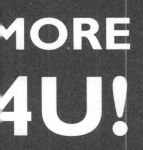

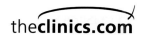

HAND CLINICS

Wrist Arthritis

GUEST EDITOR
Brian D. Adams, MD

November 2005 • Volume 21 • Number 4

SAUNDERS

An Imprint of Elsevier, Inc.
PHILADELPHIA   LONDON   TORONTO   MONTREAL   SYDNEY   TOKYO

W.B. SAUNDERS COMPANY

A Division of Elsevier Inc.

1600 John F. Kennedy Blvd. • Suite 1800 • Philadelphia, Pennsylvania 19103

http://www.theclinics.com

HAND CLINICS
November 2005
Editor: Debora Dellapena

Volume 21, Number 4
ISSN 0749-0712
ISBN 1-4160-2663-0

The ideas and opinions expressed in *Hand Clinics* do not necessarily reflect those of the Publisher. The Publisher does not assume any responsibility for any injury and/or damage to persons or property arising out of or related to any use of the material contained in this periodical. The reader is advised to check the appropriate medical literature and the product information provided by the manufacturer of each drug to be administered to verify the dosage, the method and duration of administration, or contraindications. It is the responsibility of the treating physician or other health care professional, relying on independent experience and knowledge of the patient, to determine drug dosages and the best treatment for the patient. Mention of any product in this issue should not be construed as endorsement by the contributors, editors, or the Publisher of the product or manufacturers' claims.

Hand Clinics (ISSN 0749-0712) is published quarterly by the W.B. Saunders Company. Corporate and Editorial Offices: 1600 John F. Kennedy Blvd., Suite 1800, Philadelphia, PA 19103-2899. Accounting and Circulation Offices: 6277 Sea Harbor Drive, Orlando, FL 32887-4800. Periodicals postage paid at Orlando, FL 32862, and additional mailing offices. Subscription price is $215.00 per year (U.S. individuals), $335.00 per year (U.S. institutions), $110.00 per year (US students), $245.00 per year (Canadian individuals), $375.00 per year (Canadian institutions), $135.00 (Canadian students), $275.00 per year (international individuals), $375.00 per year (international institutions), and $135.00 per year (international students). Foreign air speed delivery is included in all *Clinics* subscription prices. All prices are subject to change without notice. POSTMASTER: Send address changes to *Hand Clinics*, W.B. Saunders Company, Periodicals Fulfillment, Orlando, FL 32887-4800. **Customer Service: 1-800-654-2452 (US). From outside the US, call 1-407-345-4000. E-mail: hhspcs@harcourt.com.**

Reprints. For copies of 100 or more, of articles in this publication, please contact the Commercial Rights Department, Elsevier Inc., 360 Park Avenue South, New York, NY 10010-1710. Tel: (212) 633-3813, Fax: (212) 462-1935, e-mail: reprints@elsevier.com

Hand Clinics is covered in *Index Medicus, Current Contents/Clinical Medicine, EMBASE/Excerpta Medica,* and *ISI/BIOMED.*

Printed in the United States of America.

GUEST EDITOR

BRIAN D. ADAMS, MD, Professor of Orthopedic Surgery and Biomedical Engineering; Director of Hand and Upper Extremity Fellowship, Department of Orthopedic Surgery, University of Iowa, Iowa City, Iowa

CONTRIBUTORS

BRIAN D. ADAMS, MD, Professor of Orthopedic Surgery and Biomedical Engineering; Director of Hand and Upper Extremity Fellowship, Department of Orthopedic Surgery, University of Iowa, Iowa City, Iowa

LARS ADOLFSSON, MD, Professor, Department of Orthopaedic Surgery, University Hospital, Linkoping, Sweden

MATTHEW C. ANDERSON, MD, Fellow in Hand Surgery, Department of Orthopedic Surgery, University of Iowa, Iowa City, Iowa

ALLEN ANDREWS, BA, MPhil, Staff Research Associate, Department of Orthopaedic Surgery, University of California San Francisco, San Francisco, California

McPHERSON BEALL, MD, Hand Fellow, Department of Orthopaedic Surgery, University of California San Francisco, San Francisco, California

RICHARD A. BERGER, MD, PhD, Professor, Orthopedic Surgery and Anatomy, Mayo Clinic College of Medicine, Rochester, Minnesota

WILLIAM P. COONEY III, MD, Professor, Orthopedic Surgery, Mayo Clinic College of Medicine, Rochester, Minnesota

EDWARD DIAO, MD, Professor of Orthopaedic Surgery and Neurological Surgery; Chief, Division of Hand, Upper Extremity, and Microvascular Surgery; Medical Director, University of California San Francisco/Mount Zion Orthopaedic Faculty Practice, Department of Orthopaedic Surgery, University of California San Francisco, San Francisco, California

JOHN ELFAR, MD, Resident, Department of Orthopaedics, University of Rochester Medical Center, Rochester, New York

MATTHEW ENNA, MD, Resident, Department of Orthopaedics, Brown Medical School, Providence, Rhode Island

KEITH A. GLOWACKI, MD, Medical Director, Advanced Orthopaedic Centers; Assistant Clinical Professor, Virginia Commonwealth University, Medical College of Virginia, Richmond, Virginia

MICHAEL R. HAUSMAN, MD, Professor, Chief, Hand and Upper Extremity Service, Department of Orthopaedic Surgery, The Mount Sinai School of Medicine, New York, New York

RADFORD J. HAYDEN, PA-C, Division of Elbow, Hand, and Microsurgery, Department of Orthopaedic Surgery, University of Michigan Health Systems, Ann Arbor; Affiliate Associate Professor, College of Health Professions, Physician Assistant Studies, University of Detroit Mercy, Detroit, Michigan

DANIEL B. HERREN, MD, Handsurgery Department, Schulthess Klinik, Zurich, Switzerland

PETER HOEPFNER, MD, Assistant Professor, Department of Orthopaedic Surgery, Northwestern University Medical School, Chicago, Illinois

HAJIME ISHIKAWA, MD, Rheumatic Center, Niigata Prefectural Senami Hospital, Murakami, Japan

PETER J.L. JEBSON, MD, Associate Professor, Chief, Division of Elbow, Hand, and Microsurgery, Department of Orthopaedic Surgery, University of Michigan Health Systems, Ann Arbor, Michigan

STEVE K. LEE, MD, Assistant Professor, Hand and Upper Extremity Service, Department of Orthopaedic Surgery, The Mount Sinai School of Medicine, New York, New York

PETER M. MURRAY, MD, Associate Professor, Division of Hand and Microvascular Surgery, Department of Orthopaedic Surgery, Mayo Graduate School of Medicine, Rochester, Minnesota; Consultant, Division of Hand and Microvascular Surgery, Department of Orthopaedic Surgery; Chair, Division of Education, Mayo Clinic, Jacksonville, Florida

A. LEE OSTERMAN, MD, President, The Philadelphia Hand Center; Professor, Thomas Jefferson University Medical Center, Philadelphia, Pennsylvania

GHAZI M. RAYAN, MD, Clinical Professor of Orthopedic Surgery, Hand Surgery Section, Orthopedic Surgery Department, University of Oklahoma College of Medicine; Chairman, Hand Surgery Division, INTEGRIS Baptist Medical Center, Oklahoma City, Oklahoma

MATTHEW M. TOMAINO, MD, MBA, Professor of Orthopaedics, Chief, Division of Hand, Shoulder and Elbow Surgery, Department of Orthopaedics, University of Rochester Medical Center, Rochester, New York

H. KIRK WATSON, MD, Clinical Professor, Department of Orthopaedics, University of Connecticut Medical School, Farmington; Assistant Clinical Professor of Plastic Surgery, Yale New Haven Medical School, New Haven; and Director, Connecticut Combined Hand Surgery Fellowship, Hartford, Connecticut

ARNOLD-PETER C. WEISS, MD, Professor and Assistant Dean of Medicine (Admissions), Department of Orthopaedics, Brown Medical School, Providence, Rhode Island

RONIT WOLLSTEIN, MD, Faculty, Department of Surgery, Division of Plastic and Reconstructive Surgery, University of Pittsburgh Medical Center; University of Pittsburgh Medical Center Presbyterian and Southside Hospitals; Director of Hand Service, VA Hospital of Pittsburgh, Pittsburgh, Pennsylvania

JEFFREY YAO, MD, Assistant Professor of Orthopedics, Stanford University Medical Center, Palo Alto, California

CONTENTS

nonunion advanced collapse (SNAC) and scapholunate advanced collapse (SLAC). In the past, end-stage SLAC/SNAC arthritis generally was treated with a total wrist arthrodesis. Since the 1980s, scaphoid excision and four-corner fusion has become an increasingly popular treatment option for patients who have stage II or III SLAC/SNAC arthritis. This article (1) provides a brief overview of carpal kinematics, (2) describes the stages of SNAC and SLAC arthritis, (3) offers treatment options for SNAC/SLAC wrists, (4) reviews the surgical techniques for four-corner fusion, and (5) presents the current data supporting the use of four-corner fusion for SLAC/SNAC arthritis.

The main indications for scaphotrapeziotrapezoid (STT) fusion are STT arthritis, rotary subluxation of the scaphoid, and Kienbock disease. The results of this procedure in the literature for each indication are discussed, as are the advantages, disadvantages, and alternative procedures. This article discusses the authors' surgical technique and results. The authors believe this procedure is a viable one in specific clinical scenarios.

The correct treatment of wrist deformation in the patient who has rheumatoid arthritis has a major impact on the preservation of function of the hand. Surgical decisions should be individualized, based on the patient's needs and the future development of deformation. Partial wrist arthrodesis in rheumatoid wrists is an excellent tool to preserve stability and functional mobility in the long term. In cases of severe destruction complete wrist fusion should be considered alternatively.

In this article, proximal row carpectomy is discussed in terms of history, indications, evaluation of the appropriate patients to benefit from this so-called "salvage" procedure, and surgical alternatives to proximal row carpectomy. Focus then is placed on the surgical techniques for proximal row carpectomy and alternative treatments. Finally, expected outcomes are discussed based on salient studies in the literature.

Despite previous reports of high complication rates for limited arthrodesis procedures in the wrist, degenerative or inflammatory arthritis found isolated to the radiocarpal articulation presents the surgical option for a radioscapholunate arthrodesis to preserve some wrist motion. The purpose of this article is to review the kinematics, technique, and results of radioscapholunate arthrodesis.

This article addresses the biomechanical bases for treatment options for ulnar impaction syndrome, highlights the authors' pearls regarding examination and diagnosis, and details the surgical options, in particular, the authors' preference—arthroscopic wafer resection of the distal ulna.

CONTENTS

various inflammatory, degenerative, and post-traumatic conditions. Despite the loss of wrist motion, most patients report satisfactory functional outcomes, confirming that they are able to accomplish most daily activities of living with some adaptation and compensation. Wrist arthrodesis is an acceptable treatment approach for those patients in whom a limited arthrodesis or total wrist arthroplasty is contraindicated.

FORTHCOMING ISSUES

RECENT ISSUES

HAND CLINICS

Preface

Wrist Arthritis

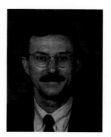

Brian D. Adams, MD
Guest Editor

Although the population is aging, demands and expectations to maintain an active lifestyle are increasing. Arguably, arthritis is the most common cause of physical debilitation and is among the top reasons for seeking medical care. Despite widespread public familiarity of available treatment for hip and knee arthritis, lack of knowledge and confusion is common not only in the lay public but also among physicians, other medical providers, and insurers regarding available treatment for upper limb arthritis. Perhaps some of this confusion relates to the higher complexity of the joints and the greater spectrum of treatment options. In addition, people have historically been more tolerant of the functional loss caused by hand and wrist arthritis, but this tendency is changing, with more people seeking out specialized care and even specific surgical procedures. It is thus imperative that health care specialists of the upper limb are knowledgeable of the pathoanatomy, clinical presentations, and surgical alternatives for arthritis. Furthermore, it is vital to our specialty that we educate other medical providers, insurers, and the public regarding our capability to substantially improve the lives of those suffering from arthritis.

By its very nature, treatment of the arthritic wrist is fascinating and challenging. The old medical adage that when multiple treatments are being used for a condition it indicates no one treatment is particularly good does not apply to the wrist. Because the wrist is a complex integrated system of joints, it requires a diversity of treatment options. In this edition of *Hand Clinics*, I have asked experts from around the world to offer their insights into the treatment of wrist arthritis. I am indebted to these experts who have provided considerable time and effort to make this a successful publication. I am confident that you will find these readings helpful to your practice. Some articles are intended to clarify and update more established procedures, whereas others introduce newer concepts and techniques. As the guest editor, it is with pride that I present this edition on a topic that has been a passion in my professional life.

Brian D. Adams, MD
Department of Orthopedic Surgery
University of Iowa Hospitals and Clinics
Lower Level, Pappajohn Pavilion
200 Hawkins Drive
Iowa City, IA 52242, USA

E-mail address: Brian-D-Adams@uiowa.edu

ELSEVIER
SAUNDERS

Hand Clin 21 (2005) 507–517

HAND CLINICS

Pisiform Ligament Complex Syndrome and Pisotriquetral Arthrosis

Ghazi M. Rayan, MD

Hand Surgery Section, Orthopedic Surgery Department, University of Oklahoma College of Medicine and INTEGRIS Baptist Medical Center, 3366 NW Expressway, Suite #700, Oklahoma City, OK 73112, USA

Pisiform ligament complex (PLC) syndrome is defined as ulnar palmar wrist pain in the vicinity of the pisiform caused by injury to components of the PLC leading to pisotriquetral (PT) joint instability with subsequent arthrosis. PT joint osteoarthritis is a degenerative joint disease involving the articular surfaces of the pisiform and triquetrum. Primary osteoarthritis of the PT joint is uncommon and many arthritic disorders of this joint are post-traumatic in nature preceded by chronic PT joint instability. PT joint osteoarthritis therefore cannot be viewed in a vacuum, because its pathophysiology overlaps and intertwines with those of other disorders. A more catholic term for arthritic conditions of this joint would be pisotriquetral arthrosis (PTA). Studying the anatomy and biomechanics of the pisiform and PT joint ligaments and reviewing the clinical variants of PLC syndrome are essential for understanding the nature of PTA.

Anatomy

In 1944 Harris [1] stated that in primates except man the pisiform has a secondary ossification center with an epiphysis, which suggests that it is analogous to the os calcis. The pisiform in humans is cartilaginous at birth and later develops one and rarely a secondary ossification center. If the secondary center is present and does not fuse to the remaining bone, an accessory ossicle develops called os pisiforme secundarium. In 1945

E-mail address: ouhsqmr@aol.com

Michelson [2] reported that the ossification of the pisiform occurs at a mean age of 8 years and 9 months and by age 12 years the bone becomes fully developed.

The pisiform is the smallest carpal bone and is located palmar to the plane of the remaining three carpal bones of the proximal carpal row. Its articulation with the triquetrum seems to be separate from other wrist articulations [3]. The pisiform is almost spherical and embedded within the flexor carpi ulnaris (FCU) tendon, thus acting as a sesamoid bone. It is the only carpal bone with one articular surface and any tendinous insertion. The pisiform receives its blood supply through the proximal and distal poles from branches of the ulnar artery. The triquetrum is pyramidal in shape and has three articular surfaces. Its palmar articular surface is the smallest, oval in shape and articulates with the pisiform. The medial wall of Guyon canal is formed by the pisiform, which is in proximity to the ulnar nerve and artery.

In 1945 Kropp [4] published a brief anatomic study that ushered in the first known modern interest in the anatomy and description of PT joint. He observed a communication between PT and radiocarpal joints in 76% of specimens. This was contradictory to descriptions by standard anatomy textbooks at the time, which implied that the PT joint has separate articulation from the wrist. Weston [5] in a brief report on postmortem arthrography confirmed this communication between the PT and wrist joints. Viegas and colleagues [6] also reported a communication between the proximal wrist joint and PT joint in 88% of cadavers dissected. Pevny and colleagues [7] described 10 soft tissue attachments to the pisiform, including the FCU tendon, extensor retinaculum, abductor digiti minimi, transverse carpal ligament (TCL), anterior carpal ligament, ulnar collateral ligament, triangular fibrocartilage complex (TFCC), pisohamate (PH) ligament, pisometacarpal (PM) ligament, and PT joint fibrous capsule. Yamaguchi and colleagues [8] identified three different anatomic types of PH and PM ligaments based on their attachment to the pisiform.

Recently Rayan and colleagues [9] coined the term pisiform ligament complex (PLC) to describe a group of ligaments that attach to the pisiform and contribute to its stability in different planes. The main ligaments that attach to the pisiform are the PM, PH, radial PT, ulnar PT, and TCL. These ligaments secure the pisiform to the triquetrum, hamate, and base of the fifth metacarpal. The fibrous tissue connecting the pisiform to the triquetrum that is often referred to as the PT joint capsule consists of the radial and ulnar PT ligaments.

Kinematics and biomechanics

The pisiform is not a mere focal point of ST attachments, rather it is a sesamoid bone that acts as a lever to enhance the function of the FCU muscle in a similar fashion to the patella and quadriceps muscle. Its attachment to the hamate through the PH ligament acts as an additional link to the triquetrohamate ligament between the proximal and distal carpal rows. The FCU tendon is the only dynamic structure that acts directly on the pisiform exerting proximally directed force. Wrist extensors and radial/ulnar deviators act indirectly by generating forces that result in pisiform displacement.

Weston [5] observed a substantial mobility of the pisiform during wrist motion and attributed this mobility to a lax capsule. Vasilas and colleagues [10] found that the PT joint space ranges from 1–4 mm in neutral wrist position and noted widening of this space with wrist flexion and its narrowing with extension. Moojen and colleagues [11] studied the pisiform kinematics and found that during extension the pisiform translates and presses against the distal part of the triquetrum but moves away from it during flexion. With radial wrist deviation the pisiform flexes while the triquetrum extends; with ulnar deviation the triquetrum shows more ulnar deviation and extension. Jameson and colleagues [12] evaluated wrists of normal volunteers fluoroscopically and

radiographically and found the pisiform has a spatial motion in relation to the triquetrum that occurs in four planes: proximal–distal (vertical gliding), anterior–posterior (gapping), uniaxial rotation (angulation), and ulnar–radial (horizontal gliding).

Pevny and colleagues [7] found that the soft tissue attachments to the pisiform were strongest distally and weakest ulnarly. No significant decrease in the stiffness of the PT joint was observed in any direction tested after transection of the TCL. Recently Rayan and colleagues [9] found the PLC to comprise primary and secondary stabilizers depending on the degree of stability provided to the pisiform and PT joint. The primary stabilizers are the PM ligament, which provides stability against proximal displacement, PH ligament against ulnar displacement, and ulnar PT ligament against radial displacement of the pisiform (Figs. 1 and 2). The radial PT ligament and TCL played a less important stabilizing role. The TCL was observed to have no attachment in the pisiform in 50% of specimens, and in the remaining 50% it was attached only to 20% of the pisiform distally. Releasing the TCL for carpal tunnel syndrome therefore should not have adverse effects on PT joint stability.

Beckers and Koebke [13] studied the mechanical strain at the PT joint and transfer of forces within the carpus. They suggested that the pisiform contributes to the stability of the ulnar column of the wrist by holding the triquetrum in a correct position and preventing its subluxation and by acting as a fulcrum while transducing powerful forearm forces to the hand. They concluded that excision of the pisiform should be

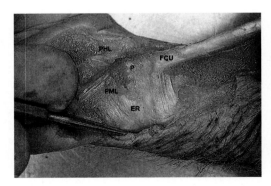

Fig. 1. Cadaver specimen showing the ulnar side of the wrist with the extensor retinaculum (ER), pisiform (P), flexor carpi ulnaris (FCU), pisohamate (PHL), and pisometacarpal (PML) ligaments.

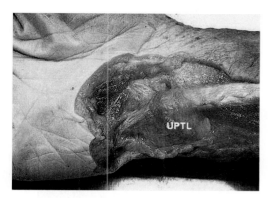

Fig. 2. The same specimen as in Fig. 1, showing the ulnar pisotriquetral ligament (UPTL) after removing the extensor retinaculum.

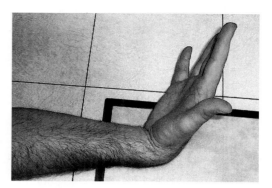

Fig. 4. Motion views for optimum viewing of the pisotriquetral joint; the forearm is positioned in 45° of supination, wrist in flexion, and thumb abducted.

reconsidered. This conclusion, however, is not substantiated by clinical studies. Studies from the author's institute suggest that the lunotriquetral ligament may be an extension of the PLC. It is yet to be determined, however, what if any adverse changes pisiform excision has on the biomechanics of the ulnar wrist.

Imaging

The radiographic technique for PT joint evaluation used at the author's institute includes at least three semilateral wrist motion views, full wrist extension with the forearm in 30° of supination (Fig. 3), neutral wrist position with 30° of supination, and full wrist flexion (active and passive optional) with 45° of supination while the thumb is fully abducted [12] (Fig. 4). These views show pisiform pathology or fractures and PTA. Also they can give the clinician insight into the pisiform motion and degree of PT joint instability (Figs. 5–8). The average normal values

for pisiform excursion, PT wedge angle, PT joint space, and PH distance can be used as parameters for comparison when instability is suspected [12]. Carpal tunnel views may visualize the pisiform from a different projection but cannot be obtained easily and are less useful than the semilateral views. Real time fluoroscopy during wrist flexion and extension with comparison to the contralateral normal side can add more information if needed about PT joint instability. Bone scan may be positive in fractures and tumors of the pisiform but is not helpful in diagnosing PTA. Trispiral tomography can delineate PT loose bodies.

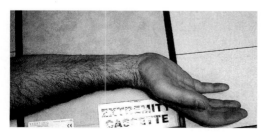

Fig. 3. Motion views for optimum viewing of the pisotriquetral joint; the forearm is positioned in 30° of supination and wrist in extension.

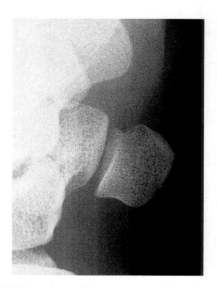

Fig. 5. The radiographic appearance of the pisotriquetral joint space in neutral wrist position.

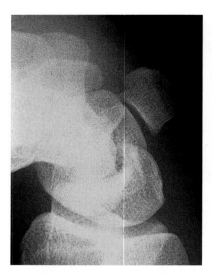

Fig. 6. The radiographic appearance of the pisotrique-tral joint space in wrist extension.

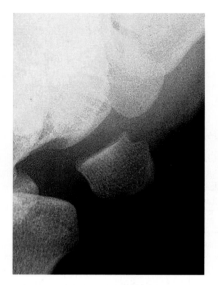

Fig. 8. The radiographic appearance of the pisotrique-tral joint space in active wrist flexion.

Theumann and colleagues [14] found in a ca-daver study that the ECU tendon sheath, fibrous capsule, and cartilaginous surfaces of the PT joint are better visualized at MR arthrography than MR imaging. The same technique allowed visual-ization of PH and PM ligaments. They concluded that this modality improves the visualization of osteoarthritis of the PT joint.

Pathology and clinical variants of pisiform ligament complex syndrome

Paley and colleagues [15] reported 16 patients with symptomatic PT joints and made correla-tions between etiologic factors and the pathologic diagnosis. They retrieved pathologic–etiologic data from 216 cases identified from the literature and organized them into four pathologic groups: primary osteoarthritis (2.3%), secondary osteoar-thritis (48.4%), other arthritides (4.7%), and FCU enthesopathy (44.6%). The most common causes were acute and chronic trauma and instability. They hypothesized that loss of integrity to the sur-rounding retinacular structures of the pisiform may lead to its instability and thus dysfunction of the joint. The following are various pathologic disorders that affect the pisiform and PT joint causing ulnar sided wrist pain. Some of these con-ditions may contribute to the development of PLC syndrome and predispose to PTA.

Congenital disorders

Congenital anomalies of the pisiform and PT joint include accessory ossicle of the pisiform, which is called os pisiforme secundarium, pisiform hamate coalition, which is often bilateral, and

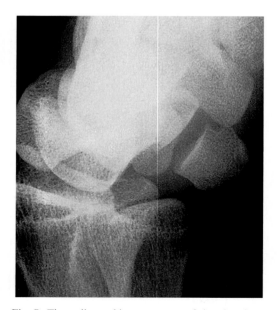

Fig. 7. The radiographic appearance of the pisotrique-tral joint space in passive wrist flexion.

congenital absence of the pisiform, which is associated with ulnar deficiency and ectrodactyly. These anomalies are rare and usually asymptomatic. Recognizing the abnormal anatomy is important to avoid misdiagnosing the condition as PTA, pisiform fracture, or scaphoid dislocation [16].

Pisiform tumors

Ganglions were described to originate from the PT joint [17] or intraosseous from the pisiform [18]. Osteoid osteoma of the pisiform also was reported, but with difficulty and delay in the diagnosis. Surgical removal of the nidus was curative in one case report [19]. Primary malignant tumors and metastatic lesions of the pisiform are extremely rare. Painful pisiform enlargement and sclerosis of the entire bone in one case report was attributed possibly to avascular necrosis. Pisiform excision did not reveal specific diagnosis but relieved the patient's symptoms [20].

Flexor carpi ulnaris tendinopathy

This probably is caused by degenerative changes within the FCU tendon near its insertion in the pisiform. Paley and colleagues [15] found that FCU enthesopathy is the cause of symptoms in 44% of patients studied who had ulnar palmar wrist pain. FCU tendinopathy, however, seldom occurs in isolation and often is associated with other conditions, especially PT instability and PTA. Diagnosing FCU tendinopathy therefore must raise the suspicion of other associated conditions.

Pisiform fracture malunion

Fractures of the pisiform can be displaced or nondisplaced or they can be extra-articular or intra-articular. Most pisiform fractures are nondisplaced, but many are intra-articular. Most pisiform fractures initially can be treated nonoperatively with splint or cast immobilization with at least short-term satisfactory results. Severely comminuted intra-articular fractures with articular cartilage damage and displaced intra-articular fractures can result later in malunion and PTA. In some cases, however, despite healing with near anatomic alignment, painful union develops and the patient continues to experience PT pain despite normal appearing radiographs. In these cases the residual pain is caused by healing with

occult malunion, malalignment of the PT joint, early PTA or associated PLC injury, and pisiform instability.

Pisiform instability

In 1948 Immerman [21] reported a case of distal pisiform dislocation and found that by 1901 there were seven such reports that antedated the discovery of radiographs. Since this publication there have been many sporadic case reports, but no series or clinical studies have been published on pisiform dislocation or its sequelae. Pisiform dislocation occurs in isolation or in association with other injuries, such as distal radius fractures [22] or hamate dislocation [23]. The mechanism of pisiform dislocation is direct force, such as a fall on the heel of the hand, or indirect force from wrist extension and FCU muscle contraction.

Two case reports described surgical treatment for acute pisiform dislocation, including open reduction and temporary internal fixation [24] and open reduction and reconstruction of the ligaments [25] with subsequent subluxation of the pisiform after both treatment modalities and post-traumatic arthritic changes in one case [25].

Recurrent dislocation of the pisiform was reported by Ishizuki [26] to occur distal to the triquetrum when the wrist was extended to 45° or more and the pisiform was reduced to proper joint congruity after wrist flexion of 55° or more. Pevny and Rayan [27] reported a case of recurrent radial dislocation of the pisiform. At surgery the pathology was attenuation of the ulnar PT ligament.

PT joint instability without dislocation is a common but unrecognized and under-reported cause of ulnar palmar wrist pain. Injuries of the PLC can be acute or chronic. There are two possible mechanisms by which acute PLC injuries occur that are similar to those of pisiform dislocation. The first is direct, caused by a fall on the outstretched hand with the force directed to the pisiform causing displacement and deformation of its ligaments but not severely enough to cause pisiform dislocation. The second is indirect, caused by wrist hyperextension with the generation of tensile forces through the ligaments, in particular the strong PH ligament or ulnar PT ligament, causing their elongation and failure. Although complete rupture of the PH ligament has not been reported, the author encountered a case of avulsion fracture of the hamulus from its base by the PH ligament caused by wrist hyperextension [28]. PT instability was reported to cause digital flexor tendon rupture [29].

Chronic PLC injuries may be a sequela of pisiform dislocation or may be caused by repetitive occupational or recreational activities. If adequate treatment or immobilization is not provided initially for acute PLC injury, this also may result in chronic pisiform instability. Conceivably any of the PLC components can be injured, but injuries to the primary stabilizers of the PT joint are probably the culprit of this joint's instability. This instability compromises the PT joint kinematics and predisposes to chondromalacia and subsequent degenerative changes. PTA is therefore an end stage on the spectrum of PLC syndrome. Pisiform instability in relation to the trapezium is not easily recognized radiographically and also was described in the literature under pisiform subluxation. Subluxation of the PT joint without pisiform dislocation was noted in 12 of 40 patients who had distal radius fracture [10]. Radiographically instability of the PT joint can be classified into three stages: I, without radiographic findings; II, with altered normal parameters (Figs. 9 and 10) with or without subluxation; and III, manifested as dislocation. Stage I radiographic instability, however. clinically can be a cause of chronic and unremitting pain.

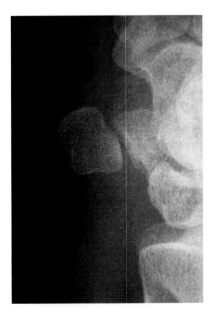

Fig. 9. Narrowing of pisotriquetral joint space while the wrist is in neutral position in a patient who has chronic instability of the pisotriquetral joint and moderate arthrosis.

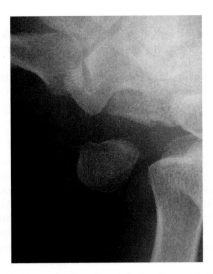

Fig. 10. The patient's radiograph showing marked widening of pisotriquetral joint space during wrist flexion.

Pisotriquetral joint loose bodies

Loose bodies may form within the PT joint or migrate from the radiocarpal joint. They may develop in the presence of a normal joint or in association with PTA. These are often cartilaginous and therefore cannot always be identified on radiographs. Tomography or MRI studies allow better visualization of these loose bodies. Treatment of symptomatic cases is by excision of the loose body or pisiformectomy if PTA is encountered during surgery.

Steinmann and colleagues [30] repotted eight patients who underwent excision of PT loose bodies; four patients reported traumatic onset of symptoms and four reported an insidious onset. Nonoperative treatment failed in all patients. Routine radiography revealed a loose body in only four patients. Trispiral tomography delineated all loose bodies. Three patients underwent loose-body excision only; five had PT joint degeneration and underwent additional pisiformectomy. All patients had pain relief and improvement in strength.

Pisotriquetral joint arthrosis

Although inflammatory arthritic conditions such as rheumatoid arthritis can affect the PT joint, they are described rarely in the literature and do not seem to be a problem to the patient. Most PT arthritic disorders are post-traumatic in nature and few are caused by primary osteoarthritis. Paley and colleagues [15] found that most cases of ulnar palmar wrist pain were caused by acute and chronic trauma and instability. Patterns of degenerative joint disease were described by Yamaguchi and colleagues [8] and Jameson and colleagues [9], both of whom reported peripheral arthritic changes in the pisiform (Fig. 11). Theumann and colleagues [14] found on cadaver wrist MR arthrography, pisiform cartilaginous lesions in 91% with a mean grade of 2.3; 50% were peripheral and 50% were global, 55% had osteophytes most often proximal, although these can be located distally or proximal and distally. Triquetral cartilaginous lesions were observed in 73% of the specimens with a mean grade of 1.6 and osteophytes were present in only 5%. FCU tendinopathy and ulnar tunnel syndrome may be associated with PTA. Takami and colleagues [31] reported attrition ruptures of the flexor digitorum profundus tendon of the little finger secondary to osteoarthritis of the PT joint. Mechanical attrition against the radial side of the pisiform was believed to be responsible for the rupture. Caroll and Coyle [32] treated 67 patients who had painful PT joints; 42 had previous traumas and 22 had associated ulnar neuropathy, particularly in those who had a history of wrist–hand fractures and subluxation or dislocation of the pisiform. Chondromalacia was present in 29 and PT joint osteoarthritis in 20 patients.

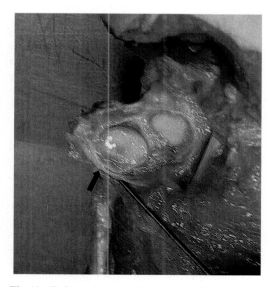

Fig. 11. Cadaver specimen showing the arthritic changes (*arrow*) in the periphery of the pisiform.

PTA is rare in young patients and may be difficult to distinguish from other ulnocarpal conditions. Trail and colleagues [33] reported PTA in 12 patients younger than 40 years of age, 10 of whom had a history of trauma.

Clinical presentation

Patients with PLC syndrome have ulnar palmar wrist pain that may radiate distally toward the hypothenar area or proximally along the FCU and ulnar aspect of the forearm. The pain can be vague and ill defined, but often is located in the hypothenar area. The pain can be deep and occasionally radiates dorsally and is aggravated by wrist motion or by using the hand in activities of daily living. In severe cases the pain may occur at rest. Examination reveals tenderness over and around the pisiform and in the soft tissues surrounding this bone. The tenderness can be elicited also over the PT joint immediately dorsal to the pisiform. Snapping or popping sensation in the ulnar palmar area may be produced with active wrist motion because of pisiform subluxation. The patient may give a history of acute injury or chronic repetitive trauma or antecedent wrist or carpal fracture.

Helal [34] described four patients whose sport involved wielding a racquet and who presented with symptoms at the hypothenar eminence caused by minor subluxation of the pisiform. In two patients there was in addition a chondromalacia of the articular cartilage of the joint, one of whom had recurrent dislocation. The physical findings in these patients were exaggerated mobility of the pisiform in axial and transverse direction.

Two useful clinical tests can be used for diagnosing PLC syndrome, in particular PTA, by which ulnar palmar pain is provoked. The first is full passive wrist extension and the second is the pisiform tracking test. The pisiform tracking test is a provocative maneuver that elicits pain and possibly crepitation and is done by flexing the wrist to relax the FCU tendon and moving the pisiform ulnarly and radially in a grinding like motion against the triquetrum. The diagnosis also can be confirmed by pain relief with local anesthetic injection of the PT joint.

Tenderness and pain proximal to the pisiform area can be caused by FCU tendopathy. In fact, diagnosing FCU tendinopathy must raise suspicion of PLC syndrome and the presence of pathology in the PT joint. In some cases of pisiform instability neurologic symptoms may be present because of associated ulnar tunnel syndrome. Closed rupture of the flexor digitorum profundus tendon of the small finger should raise the suspicion of unrecognized hamulus fracture in addition to PLC syndrome, because it was reported with PT instability and PTA [29,31]. When evaluating a patient who has suspected PLC syndrome, other wrist ligament injuries must be ruled out, such as the TFCC and those of the distal radioulnar and lunotriquetral joints. This can be accomplished by careful wrist examination to localize the area of pathology. Provocative maneuvers specific to these ligament injuries would be positive.

Treatment

Preventive measures for PLC syndrome include appropriate treatment of pisiform fractures and dislocations. Treatment of acute dislocations of the pisiform is closed reduction and splint or cast immobilization. The same treatment is appropriate for nondisplaced fractures of the pisiform. This treatment provides satisfactory outcome in most patients. Cast or rigid splint immobilization of the wrist should be attempted for all acute PLC injuries also, which may prevent the development of chronic PLC pain. Nonoperative treatment of chronic PT instability and PTA is recommended in most cases and should be used initially. This could be in the form of modifying the method of using the hand, avoiding repetitive forceful wrist flexion, and refraining from application of direct pressure on the ulnar palmar aspect of the hand. The use of weightlifting gloves can provide padding to the heel of the hand and can minimize symptoms. A period of splint immobilization, anti-inflammatory drugs, and local steroid injection may ameliorate the patient's symptoms and negate surgery. In early cases with mild or moderate PTA, local steroid injection of the PT joint together with a period of splint immobilization may bring about a long remission and surgery can be postponed or avoided.

Although repairing components of the PLC seems theoretically possible, practically it is not feasible and has not been used clinically. One reason for that trend is the apparent difficulty in diagnosing which component of the PLC is damaged. If PH ligament avulsion is encountered with a hamulus fracture, excision of the bony fragment and repair or reattachment of the ligament may provide stability and prevent residual pain and perhaps future PTA.

Surgical treatment is indicated for chronic severe PLC injuries and PTA that do not respond to nonoperative treatment measures. Pisiform excision is the universal treatment for most severe chronic cases of PLC syndrome, especially if the patient's symptoms are intolerable and nonoperative treatment measures failed. Pisiformectomy was used for various PT instabilities, including primary excision for acute pisiform dislocation [35], subluxation [18], and recurrent dislocation [26,27]. It also was used for various PT pain and arthrosis [15,32–34,36–39] with satisfactory results.

Palmieri [40] reported on 33 patients who had pisiform area pain and used pisiformectomy in 21 cases with satisfactory results. Indications for pisiformectomy were painful union and nonunion of the pisiform, PTA, and FCU tendinitis. Paley and colleagues [15] achieved satisfactory results after pisiformectomy in 8 of 16 patients who had symptomatic pisotriquetral joints.

Carroll and colleagues [32] treated 67 painful pisotriquetral joints by excision of the pisiform over a 30-year period. Forty-two patients had a previous history of trauma. Ulnar neuropathy was noted in 22 patients, particularly in those with associated wrist–hand fractures and subluxations or dislocations of the pisiform. The abductor and flexor digiti minimi and the palmar carpal ligament with their common fibrous origin were the most common compressing structures on the ulnar nerve. Chondromalacia was found in 29 and osteoarthritis in 20 PT joints. Pisiformectomy provided complete relief of localized hypothenar pain in 65 wrists with no loss of wrist motion or strength. Neurolysis produced full sensory recovery in all 22 patients and full motor recovery in 5 of 6. No late problems associated with the FCU tendon were found after pisiformectomy.

Trail and colleagues [33] reported PTA in 12 patients younger than 40 years of age who underwent pisiformectomy. They observed that patients who had a history of trauma and a positive response to intra-articular local anesthetic injection did well postoperatively. Patients who had an indefinite history and bilateral symptoms did not do so well. Trispiral tomography is the radiologic investigation of choice.

Johnston and colleagues [41] treated eight patients with PTA using pisiformectomy that produced satisfactory relief of pain after they had

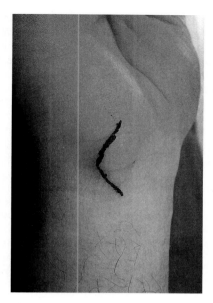

Fig. 12. The incision for pisiformectomy.

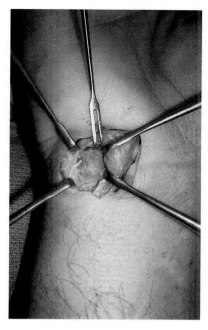

Fig. 13. Intraoperative picture showing the soft tissue confluence being retracted and the pisiform exposed.

failed to respond to splints, anti-inflammatory agents, and local steroid injection. Associated with pisotriquetral arthritis were cases of ulnar neuritis, rheumatoid arthritis, pisotriquetral joint loose bodies, and an anomalous muscle. In seven of eight patients, pisiformectomy with release of Guyon canal afforded prompt relief of pain. A palmar approach was necessary for simultaneous ulnar tunnel release and pisiform excisions. One patient with rheumatoid arthritis required a further Darrach procedure before pain was eliminated.

Belliappa and colleagues [42] reported on 12 patients with PT region pain, 11 of whom had radiologic evidence of PTA that was confirmed in the nine cases treated by pisiformectomy. Seven of these had complete relief of symptoms. Ulnar nerve symptoms were present in four patients and these also were relieved by surgery. They concluded that pisiformectomy is a useful operation for this condition, which often remains undiagnosed because of incomplete clinical and radiologic evaluation.

There is concern that pisiformectomy may result in residual pain, because it may disturb the mechanical stability it provides to the ulnar column of the wrist and loss of wrist flexion strength because of the FCU tendon insertion in the pisiform. Lam and colleagues [43] performed functional evaluation of 20 patients who had undergone pisiformectomy for PT joint dysfunction.

Fifteen patients had complete relief of symptoms and five had residual mild discomfort. Compared with the unaffected wrist, there were no significant differences in grip strength, wrist movement, static strength, and dynamic power. They concluded that pisiformectomy can be performed safely and restoration of function with a painless wrist is the expected outcome. Arner and colleagues [44] used isokinetic measurements with a strain-gauge dynamometer to assess wrist flexion strength after pisiformectomy. They found slight postoperative reduction of wrist flexion strength compared with the contralateral wrist, without clinical significance. They concluded that one should not refrain from excision of the pisiform bone for fear of considerable loss of wrist flexion strength.

Surgical technique of pisiformectomy

A 2.5-cm lateral V-shaped incision with a radially- or an ulnarly-based flap and apex at the wrist crease is planned (Fig. 12). A longer incision may be needed if ulnar nerve decompression is necessary. The skin flap is raised and the underlying pisiform and FCU tendon are identified. The ulnar nerve is dissected proximal and distal to the

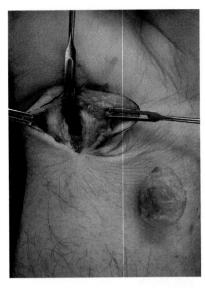

Fig. 14. The excised pisiform can be seen in the lower right corner and the preserved soft tissue confluence that can be repaired easily.

pisiform and is protected during the procedure. A soft tissue confluence can be seen overlying the pisiform. A longitudinal incision is made in the confluence and along the midportion of the FCU tendon. Careful subperiosteal dissection of the pisiform together with the soft tissue confluence is performed (Fig. 13). The PH and PM ligaments should be preserved and dissection is continued on either side of the pisiform until the articular margin is reached. The ulnar nerve is encountered against the radial aspect of the pisiform. The pisiform is excised, preserving the soft tissue confluence (Fig. 14), which is repaired meticulously together with the FCU tendon using nonabsorbable suture. This step is essential for preserving wrist flexion strength and perhaps for maintaining wrist stability. Postoperatively a dorsal splint is applied with the wrist in 20°–30° of flexion for 2 weeks. Range of motion exercises out of the splint are initiated for 2–4 weeks before discontinuing splint immobilization, depending on the patient's physical demands.

Summary

PLC syndrome is a spectrum that encompasses PLC instability and ends with PTA. Early recognition and treatment of PLC instability may disrupt its progression to PTA. The pisiform tracking test is a provocative maneuver that aids in diagnosing PLC syndrome. Pisiformectomy with preservation of the soft tissue confluence remains the treatment of choice for severe PLC syndrome that does not respond to nonoperative treatment.

References

[1] Harris H. The pisiform bone. Nature 1944;153:14.
[2] Michelson N. Studies in physical development. The ossification time of the os pisiform. Hum Biol 1945;17:142–6.
[3] Doyle JR, Botte M. Surgical anatomy of the hand and upper extremity. Philadelphia: Lippincott Williams and Wilkins; 2003.
[4] Kropp B. A note on the pisotriquetral joint. Anat Rec 1945;92:91–2.
[5] Weston WJ, Kelsey CK. Functional anatomy of the pisocuneiform joint. Br J Radiol 1973;46:692–4.
[6] Viegas SF, Patterson RM, Hokanson JA, et al. Wrist anatomy: incidence, distribution, and correlation of anatomic variations, tears, and arthrosis. J Hand Surg Am 1993;18:463–75.
[7] Pevny T, Rayan GM, Egle D. Ligamentous and tendinous support of the pisiform, anatomic and biomechanical study. J Hand Surg Am 1995;20:299–304.
[8] Yamaguchi S, Viegas SF, Patterson RM. Anatomic study of the pisotriquetral joint: ligament anatomy and cartilaginous change. J Hand Surg Am 1998; 23:600–6.
[9] Rayan GM, Jameson B, Chung K. The piso-triquetral joint: anatomic, biomechanical and radiographic analysis. J Hand Surg 2005;30:596–602.
[10] Vasilas A, Grieco RV, Bartone NF. Roentgen aspects of injuries to the pisiform bone and pisotriquetral joint. J Bone Joint Surg Am 1960;42:1317–28.
[11] Moojen TM, Snel JG, Ritt M, et al. Pisiform kinematics in vivo. J Hand Surg Am 2001;26:901–7.
[12] Jameson BH, Rayan GM, Acker RE. Radiographic analysis of pisotriquetral joint and pisiform motion. J Hand Surg Am 2002;27:863–9.
[13] Beckers A, Koebke J. Mechanical strain at the pisotriquetral joint. Clin Anat 1998;11:320–6.
[14] Theumann NH, Pfirrmann CW, Chung CB, et al. Pisotriquetral joint: assessment with MR imaging and MR arthrography. Radiology 2002;222(3): 763–70.
[15] Paley D, McMurtry RY, Cruickshank B. Pathologic conditions of the pisiform and pisotriquetral joint. J Hand Surg [Am] 1987;12(1):110–9.
[16] El-Morshidy AF, Rabia F, Mukaimi A. Bilateral asymptomatic pisiform and hamate coalition— a case report. Hand Surg 2000;5(1):57–60.
[17] Vosburgh CL, Rayan GM. Pisotriquetral joint ganglion. Orthop Rev 1994;23(5):435–6.
[18] Helal B, Vernon-Roberts B. Intraosseous ganglion of the pisiform bone. Hand 1976;8(2):150–4.

[19] Kernohan J, Beacon JP, Dakin PK, et al. Osteoid osteoma of the pisiform. J Hand Surg [Br] 1985; 10(3):411–4.

[20] Match RM. Nonspecific avascular necrosis of the pisiform bone: a case report. J Hand Surg [Am] 1980; 5(4):341–2.

[21] Immermann W. Dislocation of the pisiform. J Bone Joint Surg Am 1948;30:489–92.

[22] Ashkan K, Oconner D, Lambert S. Dislocation of the pisiform in a 9 year old child. J Hand Surg [Br] 1998;23:269–70.

[23] Gainor B. Simultaneous dislocation of the hamate and pisiform: a case report. J Hand Surg Am 1985; 10:88–90.

[24] Minami M, Yamazaki J, Ishii S. Isolated dislocation of the pisiform: a case report and review of the literature. J Hand Surg Am 1984;9:125–7.

[25] Schadel-Hopfner M, Bohringer G, Junge A. Dislocation of the pisiform bone after severe crush injury to the hand. Scand J Plast Reconstr Surg Hand Surg 2003;37(4):252–5.

[26] Ishizuki M, Nakagawa T, Itoh S, et al. Positional dislocation of the pisiform. J Hand Surg [Am] 1991;16(3):533–5.

[27] Pevny T, Rayan GM. Recurrent dislocation of the pisiform bone. Am J Orthop 1996;25:155–6.

[28] Jackson T, Rayan G. Avulsion fracture of the hamulus from clay gunshoot sport: a case report. J Hand Surg 2005;30:702–5.

[29] Corten EM, van den Broecke DG, Kon M, et al. Pisotriquetral instability causing an unusual flexor tendon rupture. J Hand Surg [Am] 2004;29(2):236–9.

[30] Steinmann SP, Linscheid RL. Pisotriquetral loose bodies. J Hand Surg [Am] 1997;22(5):918–21.

[31] Takami H, Takahashi S, Ando M, et al. Rupture of the flexor tendon secondary to osteoarthritis of the pisotriquetral joint: case report. J Trauma 1991; 31(12):1703–6.

[32] Carroll RE, Coyle MP. Dysfunction of the pisotriquetral joint: treatment by excision of the pisiform. J Hand Surg Am 1985;10:703–7.

[33] Trail IA, Linscheid RL. Pisiformectomy in young patients. J Hand Surg [Br] 1992;17(3):346–8.

[34] Helal B. Racquet player's pisiform. Hand 1978; 10(1):87–90.

[35] McCarron R, Coleman W. Dislocation of the pisiform treated with primary resection. Clin Orthop 1989;241:231–3.

[36] Krag C. Osteoarthritis of the pisotriquetral articulation. Hand 1974;6:181–4.

[37] Green DP. Pisotriquetral arthritis: a case report. J Hand Surg 1979;4:465–7.

[38] Pierre A, Le Nen D, Hu W, et al. Treatment of pisotriquetral pain by excision of the pisiform: report of fifteen cases. Chir Main 2003;22(1):37–42 [in French].

[39] Saffar P, Duek C. Piso-triquetral osteoarthritis. Thirteen case reports and review of the literature. Chir Main 2002;21(2):107–12 [in French].

[40] Palmieri T. Pisiform area pain treatment by pisiform excision. J Hand Surg 1982;7:477–80.

[41] Johnston GH, Tonkin MA. Excision of pisiform in pisotriquetral arthritis. Clin Orthop 1986;210: 137–42.

[42] Belliappa P, Burke F. Excision of the pisiform in PT osteoarthritis. J Hand Surg [Br] 1992;17:133–6.

[43] Lam KS, Woodbridge S, Burke FD. Wrist function after excision of the pisiform. J Hand Surg [Br] 2003; 28(1):69–72.

[44] Arner M, Hagberg L. Wrist flexion strength after excision of the pisiform bone. Scand J Plast Reconstr Surg 1984;18(2):241–5.

Arthroscopic Techniques for Wrist Arthritis (Radial Styloidectomy and Proximal Pole Hamate Excisions)

Jeffrey Yao, MD[a],*, A. Lee Osterman, MD[b,c]

[a]Stanford University Medical Center, 770 Welch Road, Suite 400, Palo Alto, CA 94304, USA
[b]The Philadelphia Hand Center, The Merion Building, 700 South Henderson Road,
Suite 200, King of Prussia, PA 19406, USA
[c]Thomas Jefferson University Medical Center, The Merion Building, 700 South Henderson Road,
Suite 200, King of Prussia, PA 19406, USA

Arthroscopy has achieved a greater role in hand and wrist surgery over the past 2 decades. The advent of better arthroscopic equipment and techniques has allowed the hand surgeon to complement traditional, open techniques with less invasive methods in the treatment of many common wrist disorders. The benefits of arthroscopic techniques include smaller incisions and less dissection and involvement of the surrounding soft tissues. These advantages can lead to lower morbidity, better motion, faster recovery, quicker return to work, and ultimately to higher patient satisfaction. This article details two specific arthroscopic techniques in treating wrist arthritis: radial styloidectomy and proximal pole of hamate excision.

Radial styloidectomy

Radial styloidectomy has been a standard orthopedic treatment since 1948 [1]. and recently has garnered further indications as an adjunct to other procedures around the wrist. Traditionally this procedure is performed by way of a small open incision directly over the radial styloid. Radial styloidectomy performed arthroscopically affords the benefit of visualizing exactly how much of the styloid is removed while preserving under direct vision the volar ligaments essential to the radial stability of the wrist.

Anatomy

The distal radial articular surface is made up of three surfaces and has an average total surface area of 343 mm^2. The scaphoid facet represents 46% of the total articulating surface. It is spoon-shaped and leads to the more volar radial styloid. The radial styloid is an important attachment for several ligaments that support the wrist in dorsiflexion and ulnar deviation. The lunate facet is cup shaped, articulates with the lunate, and is subject to little shear force. The lunate facet makes up approximately 43% of the total articulating surface. The triangular fibrocartilage complex [TFCC] makes up the remaining 11% of the proximal articular surface of the wrist [2,3]. The ligament anatomy of the wrist is complex, and for the purposes of this discussion, only the radially-based ligaments are discussed. The volar ligaments that derive their origin from the radial styloid include the radioscaphocapitate (RSC), radioscapholunate (RSL), and long radiolunate (LRL) ligaments. Dorsally, the radiolunotriquetral (RLT), also known as the dorsal radiocarpal (DRC) ligament also originates from the radial styloid (Figs. 1–3) [4,5]. These ligaments function to provide a sling for the scaphoid, prevent ulnar translocation of the carpus, and provide stabilization to the carpus.

Radial styloid arthritis

Jeffries showed in a cadaveric study that 27% of 138 wrists had incidental degenerative joint disease of the distal radius articular surface,

---

* Corresponding author.
E-mail address: jyao@Stanford.edu (J. Yao).

0749-0712/05/$ - see front matter © 2005 Elsevier Inc. All rights reserved.
doi:10.1016/j.hcl.2005.08.008

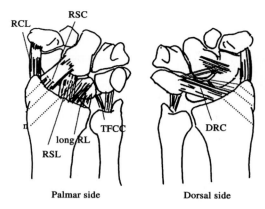

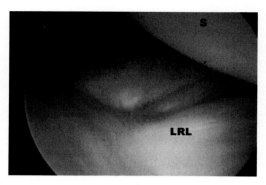

Fig. 3. Arthroscopic anatomy. RS, radial styloid; S, scaphoid; RSC, radioscaphocapitate ligament; LRL, long radiolunate ligament.

Fig. 1. Ligaments of the wrist. RCL, radiocollateral; RSC, radioscaphocapitate; RSL, radioscapholunate; long RL, long radiolunate; DRC, dorsal radiocarpal; TFCC, triangular fibrocartilage complex. (*From* Nakamura T, et al. Radial styloidectomy: a biomechanical study on stability of the wrist joint. J Hand Surg [Am] 2001;26(1):85–93; with permission.)

whereas 54% had arthritis of the proximal carpal row articular surfaces. Most commonly affected were the radial styloid and the scaphoid, respectively [6]. More common causes of radial styloid arthritis include scapholunate dissociation with advanced collapse (SLAC), scaphoid nonunion with advanced collapse (SNAC), stage IV Kienbock avascular necrosis of the lunate, and radial styloid malunion (Chauffeur fracture) [2]. Blevins showed that with SLAC wrists, the dissociation of the scaphoid from the lunate leads to instability and alteration of the kinematics and force transmission across the radiocarpal joint. Similarly, with SNAC wrists, the distal pole of the scaphoid

moves independently from the proximal pole that is still attached to the lunate. The common result from both of these entities is decreased radioscaphoid contact area, which increases point loading and leads to progressive degenerative changes along the dorsolateral aspect of the radioscaphoid joint [7].

Indications for surgery

Radial styloidectomy was described initially by Bernard in 1948 for the treatment of scaphoid nonunions [1]. Currently the most common indication for styloidectomy remains isolated radiocarpal arthritis between the scaphoid and the radial styloid. This clinical scenario is most common in cases of radial styloid malunion or *early* SLAC or SNAC wrist in which the arthritis is isolated to styloid–scaphoid impingement. Styloidectomy is also useful as an adjunct to other procedures in the treatment of Kienbock disease [8,9] and latter stage SLAC and SNAC wrist. The radial styloid may impinge on the carpus in radial deviation following triscaphe fusion [10], four-quadrant fusion [11], and proximal row carpectomy [8]. This impingement is an indication for styloidectomy, as a second procedure, or prophylactically at the time of the index procedure. Styloidectomy also may be used as an adjunct in the treatment of scaphoid nonunions, with the styloid serving as bone graft [12,13].

Treatment techniques

The standard method of performing a radial styloidectomy is by way of an open incision directly over the styloid, taking care to protect the branches of the dorsal radial sensory nerve

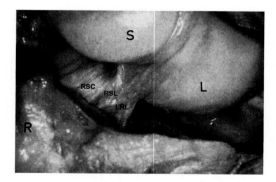

Fig. 2. Cadaveric anatomy. R, radial styloid; S, scaphoid; L, lunate; RSC, radioscaphocapitate ligament; RSL, radioscapholunate ligament; LRL, long radiolunate ligament.

[1,4,5,8–11]. Siegel showed that a short oblique osteotomy preserved the essential ligamentous attachments, thereby preserving their stabilizing function. This osteotomy sacrificed the RCL but preserved the more important RSC and LRL ligaments [4]. Similarly, Nakamura found that any styloidectomy more than 3–4 mm from the tip led to carpal instability and ultimately ulnar lunate translocation. An osteotomy of no more than 3–4 mm therefore was recommended to preserve the ligamentous attachments [5].

In isolated radiostyloid arthritis, arthroscopic styloidectomy is a viable alternative to the open procedure. Arthroscopy provides the benefits of being minimally invasive, but also the exact portion of the styloid to be resected may be visualized. This allows for the ability to visualize exactly how much styloid is to be resected while protecting the volar ligaments. Diagnostic arthroscopy may be used at the same time to evaluate any other pathology in the radiocarpal and midcarpal joints that otherwise are not detected easily with imaging studies. The styloidectomy is performed in the traction tower and using the standard wrist arthroscope from the 3-4 portal and a small 2.9- or 3.5-mm burr entering the 1-2 portal. Arthroscopy aids in visualization to ensure complete resection of the arthritic portion of the styloid (3–4 mm) without sacrificing the ligamentous support of the wrist. Also, an auxiliary portal may be helpful to allow for outflow of the debris. The diameter of the burr is a good benchmark to gauge the amount of styloid removed, and ideally this is less than 4 mm. Postoperatively these patients are placed in a volar-based short arm splint for 7–10 days, after which they return for a wound check and suture removal. Immediate wrist motion is encouraged, with protection against vigorous activity for 6 weeks (Figs. 4 and 5).

Herness reported pain relief and improved motion in patients who underwent styloidectomy in conjunction with open reduction internal fixation (ORIF) and bone grafting for scaphoid nonunion [14]. Stark also reported excellent pain relief with radial styloidectomy in patients who underwent ORIF of scaphoid nonunions, but they achieved no significant improvement of motion or grip strength [12]. Minamikawa similarly found no improvement in motion following radial styloidectomy after triscaphe fusion in cadaveric wrists [15]. Although reliable pain relief has been described following radial styloidectomy for radioscaphoid arthritis, improvement of motion is

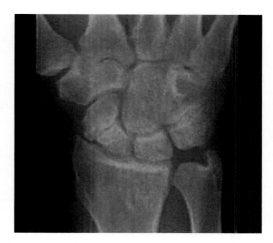

Fig. 4. PA radiograph of a wrist with radioscaphoid arthritis from a scaphoid nonunion.

therefore less reliable. This seems to be true for the open and the arthroscopic techniques.

Complications

Complications of radial styloidectomy are not unique to the open or to the arthroscopic technique. These complications include incomplete resection, loss of radial support, and excessive resection. Excessive resection leads to loss of the RSC and LRL ligaments, subsequent instability, and ultimately to ulnar translocation of the carpus [4,5,7]. Although never studied, it is likely that excessive resection is a more common complication following open styloidectomy because the amount

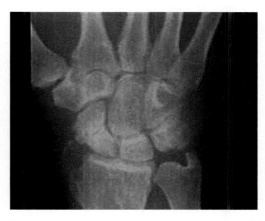

Fig. 5. PA radiograph revealing the resected radial styloid.

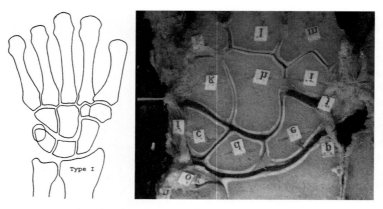

Fig. 6. Type I lunate. The hamate does not articulate with the lunate.

of resection can be monitored visually by way of the arthroscope.

Proximal pole hamate excision

Proximal pole hamate arthritis is a cause of ulnar-sided wrist pain. It is seen commonly in patients who participate in sports with ulnar-deviation loading forces, such as golf. Short of a partial wrist fusion, there is currently no adequate open procedure to treat this common problem that is often painful. Proximal pole hamate arthritis is an excellent indication for arthroscopic debridement.

Anatomy

The discussion of proximal pole of hamate arthritis must begin with a review of the pertinent anatomy. Anatomic studies reveal that lunate morphology may be classified into two types

[16,17]. Type I lunates do not articulate with the proximal pole of the hamate and are found in 35%–53% of wrists (Figs. 6–9). Type II lunates articulate with the proximal pole of the hamate by way of a distinct medial facet. This morphology accounts for 47%–65% of lunates (Figs. 7–10).

Proximal pole of hamate arthritis

Lunate morphology is important to consider, because studies have shown development of proximal pole of hamate arthritis almost exclusively in patients who have type II lunates. Incidence of arthritis in patients who have type II lunates has been reported to be as high as 44%, whereas those who have type I lunates have arthritis in only 2% [16–19]. Furthermore, Nakamura showed that 25° of ulnar deviation is the position of maximal hamatolunate joint contact. This is the position of highest contact loading of the proximal pole of

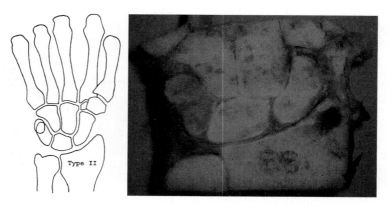

Fig. 7. Type II lunate. The proximal pole of the hamate articulates with the lunate by way of a medial lunate facet.

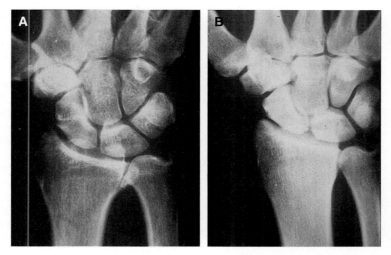

Fig. 8. PA radiographs of type I lunate (*A*) and type II lunate (*B*). Note the medial facet articulating with the hamate in *B*. (*Courtesy of* Viegas SF.)

the hamate on the medial facet of the lunate, supporting this entity as a disease of ulnar deviation [20]. Burgess and others also have shown a relationship between proximal pole of hamate arthrosis with lunatotriquetral interosseous ligament (LTIL) tears [16,18]. These entities may be parts of a continuum of ulnar-sided disease, including ulnar impaction, TFCC tears, and tearing or laxity of the ulnar extrinsic ligaments. Burgess found that 89% of patients who have proximal hamate arthrosis had a concomitant LTIL tear [16]. Harley found 91% of those patients had some degree

of LT instability. He proposed the acronym HALT (hamate arthrosis lunotriquetral ligament tear) to describe this common clinical condition [18]. Their cadaveric study, however, could not delineate whether LT instability predisposed patients who have type II lunates to develop hamate arthrosis [18].

Treatment techniques

The treatment of this common problem may be difficult. Open procedures essentially include

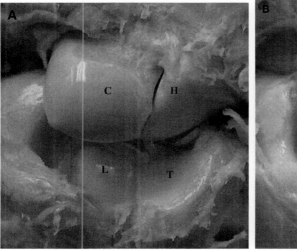
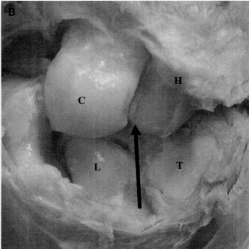

Fig. 9. Type I lunate (*A*) versus type II lunate (*B*). Notice the arthritis along the proximal pole of the hamate in (B) (*arrow*). (*Courtesy of* Viegas SF.)

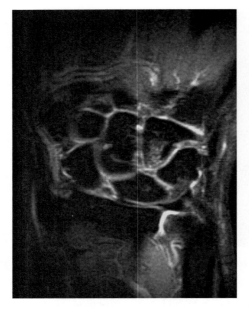

Fig. 10. Hamate arthrosis in the face of a type II lunate. Notice the medial lunate facet.

partial wrist fusion for debilitating pain. The use of arthroscopy in the excision of the proximal pole of the hamate, however, may represent more than just a temporizing measure, because excellent results have been seen in median follow-up of 4.7 years [18]. As in radial styloidectomy, arthroscopic proximal pole of hamate excision allows for the diagnosis and treatment of concomitant injuries. These include TFCC tears, LTIL tears, ulnar impaction, and any radial-side pathology. TFCC tears may be treated at the same time with debridement [21] or repair [22]. LTIL tears

may be treated with debridement, shrinkage, or pinning [18,23]. Ulnar impaction may be treated with a wafer resection [24] or with open ulnar shortening osteotomy [25]. In fact, proximal pole of hamate arthritis often is not diagnosed until the patient is in the operating room for arthroscopic treatment of any or all of the above disorders and is detected on midcarpal arthroscopy (Fig. 11A).

Proximal pole of hamate arthritis may be treated easily with arthroscopic chondroplasty, or if severe (ie, with exposed subchondral bone), with excision. The standard distraction tower and arthroscope are used. With the arthroscope in the radial midcarpal portal, a 2.9-mm burr is inserted into the ulnar midcarpal portal (Fig. 11B). An average of 2.4 mm of the proximal pole should be excised, as that has been shown to be adequate to fully unload the hamatolunate articulation while leaving loads across the triquetrohamate joint unaltered (Fig. 12) [18]. To fully excise the ulnar aspect of the proximal pole of the hamate, the portals often may be switched, with the arthroscope entering the ulnar midcarpal portal and the burr entering the radial midcarpal portal. As with the radial styloidectomy, a good rule of thumb is to excise one burr's diameter as an adequate amount of bone removed to unload the hamatolunate articulation. The postoperative care is similar to that of the radial styloidectomy as described previously.

Harley reported 86% good to excellent results with arthroscopic proximal pole of hamate excision, removing an average of 2.2 mm. Seventy-eight percent of the patients in that study had a rapid return to work. These results did not deteriorate significantly over an average of 4.7

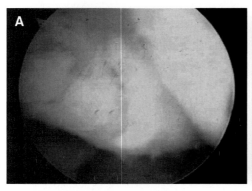

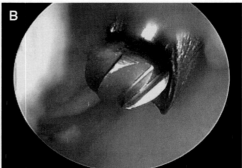

Fig. 11. (A) Arthroscopic view from the radial midcarpal portal, showing arthritis of the proximal hamate, with exposed subchondral bone. (B) A 2.9-mm burr used for the resection.

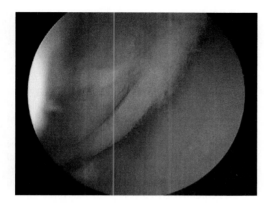

Fig. 12. Arthroscopic view of the proximal pole of the hamate following debridement.

years. The patients who did not do well had multiple concomitant injuries. That is, 100% of patients with hamate arthritis and LTIL injury alone did well, and 66% of patients with arthritis, LTIL injury, and TFCC tears did well. Only 50% of patients with combined arthritis, LTIL injury, TFCC tear, and scapholunate interosseous ligament injury achieved excellent results [18]. The rate of success of this procedure therefore depends on the number of concomitant injuries. It is a benefit of arthroscopy, however, that these diagnoses may be made at the time of the index procedure, and the patient's prognosis may be predicted. Currently, long-term studies are lacking. The consequence of excision of the proximal pole of the hamate on the midcarpal dynamics remains to be seen. The ultimate effect on the triquetrohamate articulation may be debated. At this point, however, arthroscopic proximal pole of hamate excision is an excellent minimally invasive mode of treatment for patients who have this common form of ulnar-sided wrist pain, transiently or beyond.

Summary

Over the last 2 decades, arthroscopy has assumed a greater role in the treatment of disorders of the wrist. The arthroscopic treatment of radioscaphoid arthritis and ulnar hamate impaction provides the benefits of being minimally invasive, with less morbidity, earlier motion, less recovery time, early return to work, and greater patient acceptance. Both procedures are performed easily using standard arthroscopic techniques without any significant learning curve.

Long-term studies need to be performed to determine the exact clinical sequelae of excision of the proximal pole of the hamate, specifically on the biomechanics of the triquetrohamate articulation.

References

[1] Watson HK, Black DM. Instabilities of the wrist. Hand Clin 1987;3(1):103–11.

[2] Linscheid KL. Kinematic considerations of the wrist. Clin Orthop Rel Res 1986;202:27–39.

[3] Siegel DB, Gelberman RH. Radial styloidectomy: an anatomical study with special reference to radiocarpal ligamentous morphology. J Hand Surg [Am] 1991;16A:40–4.

[4] Nakamura T, Cooney WP, Lui WH, et al. Radial styloidectomy: a biomechanical study on stability of the wrist joint. J Hand Surg [Am] 2001;26(1):85–93.

[5] Jeffries AO, Craigen MA, Stanley JK. Wear patterns of the articular cartilage and triangular fibrocartilaginous complex of the wrist: a cadaveric study. J Hand Surg [Br] 1994;19(3):306–9.

[6] Blevins AD, Light TR, Jablonsky WS, et al. Radiocarpal articular contact characteristics with scaphoid instability. J Hand Surg [Am] 1989;14(5):781–90.

[7] Barnard L, Stubbins SG. Styloidectomy of the radius in the surgical treatment of non-union of the carpal navicular: a preliminary report. J Bone Joint Surg 1948;30A:98–102.

[8] Lin HH, Stern PJ. 'Salvage' procedures in the treatment of Kienböck's disease: proximal row carpectomy and total wrist arthrodesis. Hand Clin 1993; 9:521–6.

[9] Watson HK, Ryu J, DiBella A. An approach to Kienböck's disease: triscaphe arthrodesis. J Hand Surg [Am] 1985;10A:179–87.

[10] Rogers WD, Watson HK. Radial styloid impingement after triscaphe arthrodesis. J Hand Surg [Am] 1989;14A:297–301.

[11] Watson HK, Weinzweig J, Guidera PM, et al. One thousand intercarpal arthrodeses. J Hand Surg [Br] 1999;24(3):307–15.

[12] Stark HH, Rickard TA, Zemel NP, et al. Treatment of ununited fractures of the scaphoid by iliac bone grafts and Kirschner-wire fixation. J Bone Joint Surg 1988;70A:982–91.

[13] Ruch DS, Chang DS, Poehling GG. The arthroscopic treatment of avascular necrosis of the proximal pole following scaphoid nonunion. J Arthrosc Rel Res 1998;14(7):747–52.

[14] Herness D, Posner MA. Some aspects of bone grafting for non-union of the carpal navicular: analysis of 41 cases. Acta Orthop Scand 1977;48(4):373–8.

[15] Minamikawa Y, Peimer CA, Yamaguchi T, et al. Ideal scaphoid angle for intercarpal arthrodesis. J Hand Surg [Am] 1992;17(2):370–5.

[16] Burgess RC. Anatomic variations of the midcarpal joint. J Hand Surg [Am] 1990;15A:129–31.

[17] Viegas SF, Wagner K, Patterson R, et al. Medial (hamate) facet of the lunate. J Hand Surg [Am] 1990;15A:564–71.

[18] Harley BJ, Werner FW, Boles SD, et al. Arthroscopic resection of arthrosis of the proximal hamate: a clinical and biomechanical study. J Hand Surg [Am] 2004;29(4):661–7.

[19] Thurston AJ, Stanley JK. Hamato-lunate impingement: an uncommon cause of ulnar-sided wrist pain. Arthroscopy 2000;16:540–4.

[20] Nakamura K, Beppu M, Patterson RM, et al. Motion analysis in two dimensions of radial-ulnar deviation of type I versus type II lunates. J Hand Surg 2000;25A:877–88.

[21] Minami A, Ishikawa J, Suenaga N, et al. Clinical results of treatment of triangular fibrocartilage complex tears by arthroscopic debridement. J Hand Surg [Am] 1996;21A:406–11.

[22] Trumble TE, Gilbert M, Vedder N. Isolated tears of the triangular fibrocartilage: management by early arthroscopic repair. J Hand Surg [Am] 1997;22A:57–65.

[23] Viegas SF, Patterson RM, Hokanson JA, et al. Wrist anatomy; incidence, distribution and correlation of anatomic variations, tears, and arthrosis. J Hand Surg [Am] 1993;18A:463–75.

[24] Tomaino MM, Weiser RW. Combined arthroscopic TFCC debridement and wafer resection of the distal ulna in wrists with triangular fibrocartilage complex tears and positive ulnar variance. J Hand Surg [Am] 2001;26A:1047–52.

[25] Chun S, Palmer AK. The ulnar impaction syndrome: follow-up of ulnar shortening osteotomy. J Hand Surg [Am] 1993;18A:46–53.

Hand Clin 21 (2005) 527–530

Arthroscopic Synovectomy in Wrist Arthritis

Lars Adolfsson, MD

Department of Orthopaedic Surgery, University Hospital 581, 85 Linkoping, Sweden

Surgical synovectomy was described more than one hundred years ago and later became a widely accepted method to reduce symptoms in arthritic joints during the latter half of the twentieth century. The advent of arthroscopy and specific motorized shaver systems enabled percutaneous synovectomy; first popularized in the knee joint during the 1980s. Later the technique was used in the treatment of different types of arthritic diseases and its use has been described in most peripheral joints of the body.

Synovectomy can reduce pain and swelling and improve joint function for a considerable time, but in most cases the effect is ultimately transitory, with recurrence depending on the activity of the underlying cause of the arthritis. Some have claimed that synovectomy in rheumatoid arthritis can have a positive, long-lasting effect and perhaps even halt further joint deterioration [1–7]. This has been based on anecdotal reports, however, and has not been substantiated in larger series [8,9]. Arthroscopic synovectomy of the wrist was described around 1990 [10], and shortly thereafter the first clinical results were reported [11]. There are still few studies presenting results after this procedure and no studies using control groups or a randomized design. The published short and intermediate term results, however, suggest that in patients who have rheumatoid arthritis a marked reduction of pain and an increased function can be achieved [11–14].

During the last decade, improvement in and increased specification of medications for patients who have rheumatoid arthritis has reduced the need for synovectomies, and the author's department has experienced a marked decrease in the number of these procedures.

There are still occasions, however, when arthroscopic synovectomy is indicated.

Indications

Rheumatoid arthritis

The main indication for arthroscopic synovectomy is for rheumatoid arthritis in patients for whom pharmacologic treatment has not been tolerated or sufficiently effective to reduce joint synovitis. All patients who are considered for surgery should have had at least one intra-articular steroid injection and should have had persistent joint synovitis for more than 6 months. The patient typically presents with a tender, spongy swelling dorsally over the radiocarpal joint. Palpable synovitis around the ulnar styloid and extensor carpi ulnaris (ECU) tendon is common and may extend over the scaphotrapeziotrapezoidal (STT) joint. Range of motion and grip strength usually is reduced, but true joint stiffness may be difficult to assess, because tendon involvement often contributes to reduced motion.

The author has found that if marked arthritic changes were present at the time of surgery, progression was substantially more rapid than in patients who had less severe changes [12]. Only a small number of patients with radiographic changes corresponding to grade III and IV according to the staging system by Larsen, Dale, Eek (LDE-index) [15] benefited from the surgery. Arthroscopic synovectomy therefore is now recommended only for patients who have radiographic changes of grade 0-II on the LDE index.

Patients who have juvenile rheumatoid arthritis (JRA) have been treated similarly, but the author has no experience in patients younger than 17 years of age. Previous studies on open synovectomy in patients who have JRA indicate that

E-mail address: Lars.Adolfsson@lio.se

hand.theclinics.com

the results do not differ from those in adult rheumatoid arthritis [16].

Patients who require extensive open wrist surgery are not candidates for arthroscopic synovectomy, but the author has combined it successfully with other procedures, such as tenosynovectomy, carpal tunnel release, fusion of thumb joints, reconstruction of extensor tendon ruptures, and triangular fibrocartilage complex (TFCC) reinsertion. The minor surgical trauma inflicted by the arthroscopic procedure has not seemed to affect the outcome of the other procedures.

Systemic lupus erythematosus, psoriatic arthropathy, and postinfectious monoarthritis

To the author's knowledge, no publications have reported the use of arthroscopic synovectomy of the wrist in these diseases and the indications remain unclear.

Joint afflictions in systemic lupus erythematosus (SLE) may involve the wrist, and in initial stages a wrist synovitis may be present. The clinical picture in early cases may resemble rheumatoid arthritis, and the author has used arthroscopic synovectomy in a small number of patients who have joint synovitis.

Postinfectious monoarthritis, often referred to as reactive arthritis, may occur after bacterial and viral infections. In patients who have longstanding symptoms refractory to conservative treatment, arthroscopic synovectomy has been found beneficial.

A small number of patients who have psoriatic arthropathy have been treated with arthroscopic synovectomy, but because the synovitis is less pronounced and there is a tendency for ankylosis with this disease, the results have not been encouraging and the procedure presently is not recommended for this disease.

Theoretically arthroscopic synovectomy can be used in any kind of synovial disease that is amenable for resection. As in large joints, pigmented villonodular synovitis, hemophilia and benign tumors have been treated. In the rare instance that these types of diseases affect the wrist joint, arthroscopic synovectomy may be considered.

In rare forms of arthritic diseases the indication for surgery should always be discussed with a rheumatologist.

Septic arthritis

Arthroscopic management of septic arthritis has been shown to yield good results in the knee and shoulder [17–19]. The technique has been suggested for the wrist, but no results have been published [20,21]. The author has successfully treated septic arthritis with arthroscopic synovectomy in five patients. All of the author's patients were treated initially with aspiration and lavage of the radiocarpal joint, combined with systemic antibiotics, but the patients failed to improve sufficiently during the following 48 hours. The arthroscopic procedure included biopsy for cultures, repeat lavage, and resection of inflamed synovium in the radiocarpal and midcarpal spaces.

Osteoarthritis

Osteoarthritis with minimal radiographic changes and pronounced synovitis is uncommon but possibly may benefit from arthroscopic synovectomy. Patients who have localized degenerative changes, such as those occurring at the STT joint, ulnar impaction syndrome, and radioscaphoid arthritis, often are treated with synovectomy but in combination with a resectional arthroplasty. Radial plica is a separate entity in which a hypertrophy of synovium over the radial styloid may impinge between the scaphoid and the styloid, producing localized pain and snapping. It may be confused with de Quervain disease. Arthroscopic resection of the fibrotic and hypertrophic synovium is successful for these patients.

Post-traumatic synovitis

In the author's experience, longstanding synovitis following a wrist trauma indicates an intra-articular pathology, such as ligament or cartilage lesions. Following intra-articular fractures or previous surgery the synovitis can be associated with arthrofibrosis interfering with range of motion, and in these cases synovectomy, removal of adhesions, and occasionally capsular release can improve joint mobility significantly.

Technique

Standard techniques and instrumentation for wrist arthroscopy are used [11,22–25]. A conventional traction device with finger traps is used, but the amount of traction may have to be reduced in rheumatoid patients with affected finger joints. The author also applies finger traps to all fingers to distribute the load as much as possible. Because these patients frequently have increased laxity in the wrist, only mild traction is needed.

Continuous irrigation is necessary and is obtained preferably with an automatic pressure regulated pump; however, close observation for excessive extravasation is mandatory. Passive infusion from an elevated bag of saline solution through a separate inflow cannula is possible, but this makes regulation of suction more difficult. The radiocarpal joint normally is accessed by way of the 3-4 and 6R portals, and the midcarpal space through radial and ulnar midcarpal portals. In cases with synovitis in the STT joint, a separate portal is established. In rare instances the 6U, 1-2, and distal radioulnar joint (DRUJ) portals have been used. A 3.5-mm shaver is preferred; occasionally a 2-mm shaver is used, but the smaller diameter shaver is less effective for synovectomy. Recently thermocoagulation is preferred because it is efficient and reduces bleeding that can obscure visualization. In addition, the small diameter, flexible probes facilitate access to all parts of the joints. No adverse effects have been observed. The arthroscope and shaver or electrode must be alternated between the portals to reach all parts of the joint.

In arthritic joints the synovitis typically is localized around the radial styloid, the radioscapholunate ligament, in the ulnar prestyloid recess, and dorsoulnar underneath the sixth extensor tendon compartment. The midcarpal space often is less affected, but when present the synovitis often is distributed dorsoulnar, volarly under the capitohamate joint, and in the STT joint.

Particularly with rheumatoid arthritis, synovitis may be found in the DRUJ. In these cases there is often an increased laxity in the DRUJ capsule and the TFCC. A central defect in the horizontal portion of the TFCC then is usually present. After trimming the edges of the defect, the synovectomy may be done through the defect from the 6R portal. If accessibility is inadequate, a separate DRUJ portal immediately proximal to the TFCC can be used for the shaver while viewing from the radiocarpal joint.

Postoperatively a light bandage is applied that allows gentle motion. At 10-12 days the arthroscopy portals normally are healed sufficiently to advance activity. An exercise program is prescribed if recovery of motion is difficult.

Arthroscopic synovectomy in rheumatoid wrists with no or mild radiographic changes has been reported to reduce pain and improve function, range of motion, and grip strength in short and intermediate term follow-ups [11–14].

Although the designs of the published studies do not allow definite conclusions on the efficacy of the procedure, the data suggest that a long period of increased comfort can be expected in patients who have rheumatoid arthritis. In a recent follow-up study, the author interviewed 18 patients 12–15 years after arthroscopic synovectomy and found that only 1 patient had undergone additional surgery in the same wrist (unpublished data). Six patients regarded themselves as free from wrist symptoms, seven had mild symptoms such as slight weakness and a sensation of instability, and four had moderate pain and stiffness.

Only anecdotal reports on few patients have been published on arthroscopic synovectomy in other forms of arthritis. The author's experience indicates that in patients who have JRA, SLE, reactive arthritis, and septic arthritis, the results are good, but the procedure cannot be recommended in patients who have psoriatic arthropathy.

In patients who have osteoarthritis the effect of a synovectomy is probably short-term and there are no published results to support its use as an isolated treatment. It may be considered, however, as an adjunct to a resection arthroplasty or other procedures addressing the underlying cause of the synovitis.

In post-traumatic synovitis and arthrofibrosis the synovectomy and removal of intra-articular adhesions can improve mobility and reduce pain markedly. The procedure was advocated by Osterman in 1999 [26], but no specific peer-reviewed study has reported the results of this procedure.

In one patient the author has seen a synovial fistula that required excision 4 weeks after synovectomy, but the author has not had any other complications, and no reports on complications after arthroscopic synovectomy of the wrist were found in the literature.

Summary

Arthroscopic synovectomy is a safe outpatient procedure with minimal postoperative morbidity. In patients who have rheumatoid arthritis and possibly also in patients who have JRA, SLE, and postinfectious arthritis, a long period of increased comfort and improved function can be anticipated. The procedure may be considered in post-traumatic cases with joint contracture and as an adjunct to other measures for certain osteoarthritic disorders. In patients who have septic arthritis with insufficient clinical improvement after systemic antibiotics and lavage, arthroscopic synovectomy seems advantageous.

References

[1] Aschan W, Moberg E. A long-term study on the effect of early synovectomy in rheumatoid arthritis. Bull Hosp Joint Dis Orthop Inst 1984;44:106–21.

[2] Böhler N, Lack N, Schwägerl W, et al. Late results of synovectomy of wrist, MP and PIP joints: multicenter study. Clin Rheumatol 1985;4:23–5.

[3] Ishikawa H, Ohno O, Hirohata K. Long-term results of synovectomy in rheumatoid patients. J Bone Joint Surg 1986;68A:198–205.

[4] Jensen CM, Poulsen S, Östergren M, et al. Early and late synovectomy of the knee in rheumatoid arthritis. Scand J Rheumatol 1991;20:127–31.

[5] Matsui N, Taneda Y, Ohta H, et al. Arthroscopic versus open synovectomy in the rheumatoid knee. Int Orthop 1989;13:17–20.

[6] Pahle JA, Kvarnes L. Shoulder synovectomy. Ann Chir Gynaecol 1985;74(Suppl 198):37–9.

[7] Vahvanen V, Pätiälä H. Synovectomy of the wrist in rheumatoid arthritis and related diseases. Arch Orthop Trauma Surg 1984;102:230–7.

[8] Arthritis Foundation Committee on Evaluation of Synovectomy. Multi-center evaluation of synovectomy in the treatment of rheumatoid arthritis: report of results at the end of three years. Arthritis Rheum 1977;20:765–71.

[9] Arthritis and Rheumatism Council and British Orthopaedic Association. Controlled trial of synovectomy of knee and metacarpophalangeal joints in rheumatoid arthritis. Ann Rheum Dis 1976;35:437–42.

[10] Roth JH, Poehling GG. Arthroscopi "-ectomy" surgery of the wrist. Arthroscopy 1990;6:141–7.

[11] Adolfsson L, Nylander G. Arthroscopic synovectomy of the rheumatoid wrist. J Hand Surg 1993;18B:92–6.

[12] Adolfsson L, Frisén M. Arthroscopic synovectomy of the rheumatoid wrist—a 3.8 year follow-up. J Hand Surg 1997;22B:711–3.

[13] Park MJ, Ahn JH, Kang JS. Arthroscopic synovectomy of the wrist in rheumatoid arthritis. J Bone Joint Surg 2003;85B:1011–5.

[14] Wei N, Delauter SK, Beard S, et al. Office-based arthroscopic synovectomy of the wrist in rheumatoid arthritis. Arthroscopy 2001;17:884–7.

[15] Larsen A, Dale K, Eek M. Radiographic evaluation of rheumatoid arthritis and related conditions by standard reference films. Acta Radiol 1977;18:481–91.

[16] Hanff G, Sollerman C, Elborgh R, et al. Wrist synovectomy in rheumatoid arthritis. Scand J Rheumatol 1990;19:280–4.

[17] Jerosch J, Prymka M. Arthroscopic therapy of septic arthritis. Surgical technique and results. Unfallchirurgie 1998;101:454–60.

[18] Thiery JA. Arthroscopic drainage in septic arthritides of the knee: a multi-center study. Arthroscopy 1989;5:65–9.

[19] Wirtz DC, Marth M, Miltner O, et al. Septic arthritis of the knee in adults: treatment by arthroscopy or arthrotomy. Int Orthop 2001;25:239–41.

[20] Bain GI, Roth JH. The role of arthroscopy in arthritis. Hand Clin 1995;11:51–8.

[21] Parisien JS, Shaffer B. Arthroscopic management of pyarthrosis. Clin Orthop 1992;275:243–7.

[22] Botte MJ, Cooney WP, Linscheid RL. Arthroscopy of the wrist: anatomy and technique. J Hand Surg [Am] 1989;14A:313–6.

[23] Roth JH. Hand instrumentation for small joint arthroscopy. Arthroscopy 1988;4:126–8.

[24] Whipple TL, Marotta JJ, Powell JH. Techniques of wrist arthroscopy. Arthroscopy 1986;2:244–52.

[25] Whipple TL. Powered instruments for wrist arthroscopy. Arthroscopy 1988;4:290–4.

[26] Osterman AL. Wrist arthroscopy: operative procedures. In: Green DP, Hotchkiss RN, Pederson WC, editors. Green's operative hand surgery. Philadelphia: Churchill Livingstone; 1999. p. 207–22.

Scaphoid Excision with Four-Corner Fusion

Matthew Enna, MD[a], Peter Hoepfner, MD[b],
Arnold-Peter C. Weiss, MD[a],*

[a]Department of Orthopaedics, Brown Medical School, University Orthopedics,
2 Dudley Street, Suite 200, Providence, RI 02905, USA
[b]Department of Orthopaedic Surgery, Northwestern University Medical School,
303 East Chicago Avenue, Chicago, IL 60611, USA

The scaphoid is an important anatomic and biomechanical link between the proximal and distal carpal rows [1]. This is elucidated by two scaphoid injury models—scaphoid nonunion advanced collapse (SNAC) and scapholunate advanced collapse (SLAC). In the past, end-stage SLAC/SNAC arthritis generally was treated with a total wrist arthrodesis [2]. Since the 1980s, scaphoid excision and four-corner fusion has become an increasingly popular treatment option for patients who have stage II or III SLAC/SNAC arthritis. This article (1) provides a brief overview of carpal kinematics, (2) describes the stages of SNAC and SLAC arthritis, (3) offers treatment options for SNAC/SLAC wrists, (4) reviews the surgical techniques for four-corner fusion, and (5) presents the current data supporting the use of four-corner fusion for SLAC/SNAC arthritis.

Carpal kinematics

In the uninjured wrist, the lunate maintains a neutral position between the distal radius and capitate by balancing the counter forces created by the scapholunate and lunotriquetral ligaments. The scapholunate ligament has a flexion moment resulting from flexion of the scaphoid between the distal radius and trapezium. The lunotriquetral ligament has an extension moment resulting from the triquetrum being extended relative to the

lunate. The balance of the lunate between ligamentous counter forces was termed the concertina effect by Fisk in 1970 [3]. Scaphoid fracture and scapholunate incompetence disrupt the normal intercalation between scaphoid and lunate, thus enabling extension of the lunate under the guidance of the intact lunotriquetral ligament. This has been coined dorsal intercalated instability (DISI) [4]. A corollary of this pathology is the increase in scaphoid flexion resulting from the separation of the scaphoid from the influence of the lunotriquetral ligament [5]. During the progression of SNAC/SLAC arthritis, changes in scaphoid shape, volume, and position lead to an increased load burden for the capitate, which responds by gradually migrating between the lunate and scaphoid.

A functional range of wrist motion allows one to perform activities of daily living, including dressing, eating, and personal hygiene. The research of Brumfield and Champoux indicates that the functional range of wrist motion is 10° of flexion and 35° of extension [6]. Palmer and colleagues described a functional range from 5° of flexion to 30° of extension [7]. Ruby and colleagues used cadaveric specimens to research the mean wrist flexion/extension arc [8]; their study yielded a mean value of 112°. Linscheid's research arrived at a value of 150° [9]. The effect of limited intercarpal arthrodesis on wrist range of motion was examined by Gellman and colleagues, who used in vitro analysis to determine that 63%–70% of wrist flexion occurs at the radiocarpal joint and 30%–36% occurs at the midcarpal joint [10]. The study predicts retention of 64% of the flexion–extension arc after four-corner fusion [10,11].

---

* Corresponding author.
E-mail address: apcweiss@brown.edu
(A-P.C. Weiss).

SLAC/SNAC staging

In Watson's analysis of more than 4000 wrist radiographs, 95% of all the degenerative wrist arthritis involved the scaphoid. SLAC arthritis is the most common form of noninflammatory wrist arthritis [12]. As a result of scapholunate ligament insufficiency, the scaphoid flexes and loses its normal articular congruence with the distal radius scaphoid fossa. This incongruence leads to three stages of progressive degenerative change. The SLAC wrist pattern also may be seen in uncollapsed Kienböck disease, Preiser disease, and after a distal radius fracture involving the radioscaphoid fossa [13]. Stage I SLAC involves degeneration of the radial styloid–scaphoid articulation. Stage II includes the entire radioscaphoid joint. Stage III involves capitolunate degeneration. In general, the radiolunate articulation is spared in SLAC arthritis.

Between 5% and 10% of scaphoid fractures result in nonunion [14]. Delayed diagnosis, fracture displacement, fracture location, improper immobilization, and wrist instability may factor into this rate of nonunion [3,15–20]. Scaphoid nonunion leads to a series of degenerative changes that are similar to but distinct from SLAC arthritis. Research by Mack [14] and Ruby [21] elucidated the degenerative progression seen in SNAC arthritis. In general, scaphoid nonunion cystic changes are seen one decade after fracture; radioscaphoid degeneration is evident after two decades; and pancarpal arthritis is apparent in the third decade after injury [14,21]. SNAC arthritis progression depends on several variables, including fracture type, displacement, and stability. Some investigators report that scaphoid nonunion leads to degenerative wrist arthritis in 100% of cases [21]. Similar to SLAC arthritis, stage I SNAC involves the radial styloid–scaphoid joint. Stage II includes progressive degeneration of the radioscaphoid articulation and scaphocapitate degeneration. Stage III involves capitolunate degeneration and progression of the radioscaphoid and scaphocapitate degeneration. The proximal radioscaphoid and radiolunate joints generally are spared of degenerative change.

Treatment options

Conservative measures for SLAC/SNAC wrists include activity modification, splint immobilization, steroid injection, and NSAIDs. Surgical measures should be considered when wrist pain is refractory to these conservative measures. Surgical options include total or partial wrist arthrodesis, proximal row carpectomy, distraction arthroplasty, and total wrist arthroplasty [22–24]. Historically, degenerative conditions of the wrist were treated with a total wrist arthrodesis—a procedure that provides pain relief at the expense of all wrist joint motion. Thornton reported the first use of limited wrist arthrodesis in 1924 [25], after successfully fusing the scaphoid, lunate, capitate, and hamate. The arthrodesis of the lunate, capitate, hamate, and triquetrum since has come to be known as a four-corner fusion. The biomechanical principle behind scaphoid excision and four-corner fusion is that wrist motion occurs through the preserved radiolunate and ulnocarpal joints. Including the hamate and triquetrum in the fusion mass has been shown to provide a higher fusion rate without sacrificing further motion [26].

The optimal surgical management of SLAC/SNAC wrists depends on several factors, including patient age, activity level, occupation, and stage of degeneration. Preoperative radiographs are imperative to assess the degree of wrist degeneration and to measure the DISI deformity requiring surgical correction. Stage I SLAC/SNAC wrists are best treated with radial styloid excision (with or without scaphoid fixation or bone grafting for scaphoid nonunions). Stage II treatment options include proximal row carpectomy (PRC), four-corner fusion with radial styloidectomy, and four-corner fusion with scaphoid excision. Stage III options are four-corner fusion with scaphoid excision or total wrist arthrodesis. PRC is not an option for stage III because of capitolunate joint involvement.

Contraindications for four-corner fusion in SLAC/SNAC wrists include radiolunate articular degeneration and ulnar carpal translation (usually resulting from long radiolunate ligament insufficiency), which disrupts the normal congruity of the radiolunate joint and hastens its degeneration. Total wrist arthrodesis is the procedure of choice in these cases.

Surgical technique

As described by Watson [27], four-corner fusion can be approached through a dorsal transverse incision distal to the radial styloid level. Use caution to avoid transection and overzealous retraction of the superficial branch of the radial nerve. The extensor carpi radialis longus and brevis and the extensor pollicis longus are identified and retracted, followed by scaphoid removal. The long radiolunate ligament must be preserved. A transverse capsular incision then is made at the capitolunate joint. A rongeur is used to remove the cartilaginous articulations between the lunate, capitate, hamate, and triquetrum. Next, cancellous bone is interposed between joint surfaces to enhance fusion. K-wires or staples then are placed between the capitate and lunate, triquetrum and lunate, hamate and lunate, and triquetrum and hamate (Fig. 1). Further bone graft is added after internal fixation [28]. As originally described by Watson, a Silastic scaphoid implant replaced the degenerative scaphoid. This practice was terminated as a result of implant malrotation and particulate synovitis [13].

A recent advance in four-corner fusion is the Spider plate (KMI; San Diego, CA), a conical, no-profile plate that is seated below the dorsal surface of the carpus (Fig. 2). The surgical approach is a 7-cm longitudinal incision centered over the dorsum of the carpus. Crossing branches of the superficial branch of the radial nerve are identified and protected. The extensor carpi radialis longus and brevis are freed from the dorsal wrist capsule and retracted radially. The extensor pollicis longus is transposed radially (Fig. 3). The extensor digitorum communis and extensor indicis proprius are retracted ulnarly. The posterior interosseous nerve then is identified and resected. This is followed by a T-shaped capsulotomy or a ligament-sparing dorsal capsulotomy described by Berger [28] (Fig. 4).

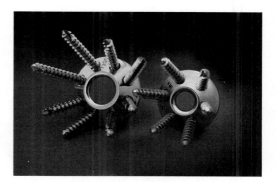

Fig. 2. The Spider and Mini-Spider plates used for limited intercarpal fusions (Courtesy of Kinetikos Medical, Inc., Carlsbad, California.)

Scaphoid excision may be facilitated by placing a joystick through the longitudinal axis of the scaphoid. A 3.2-mm drill bit is used to create bicortical drill holes; a 3.5-mm tap then is passed through the drill holes. The joystick technique allows for scaphoid manipulation as the surrounding soft-tissue attachments are released with a scalpel. The underlying volar carpal ligaments must be retained (Fig. 5).

The next step is to expose the lunate, capitate, hamate, and triquetrum, followed by correction of any carpal instability pattern (typically DISI) with Kirschner wires directed as volarly as possible (Fig. 6). Joysticks also may be of benefit in correcting a DISI deformity. Linscheid described a novel approach for reducing DISI deformity with fluoroscopy [29]. After achieving neutral alignment between radius and lunate with wrist flexion and ulnar deviation, a 0.0625-inch Kirschner wire is drilled through the dorsal distal radius into the lunate [29]. Fusion of the lunate in slight flexion relative to the capitate may provide greater wrist extension as proposed by Cohen and Kozin, whose patients had an average of 45° of extension versus an average of 31° reported in the literature [30]. After reducing any carpal instability, provisional four-corner stabilization is achieved by drilling a Kirschner wire across the capitate and triquetrum.

The articulations between the four carpal bones then are denuded to cancellous bone with a rongeur (Fig. 7). Next, the Spider rasp is centered over the four-corner junction; it rasps flush to the dorsum of the carpus, enabling recession of the Spider plate (Fig. 8). When fusing a type II lunate, the rasp should be centered at the lunate–hamate articulation [31]. The denuded

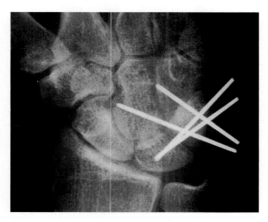

Fig. 1. Anteroposterior (AP) radiograph demonstrating fixation of the fusion using Kirschner wires (Courtesy of Arnold-Peter C. Weiss, MD.)

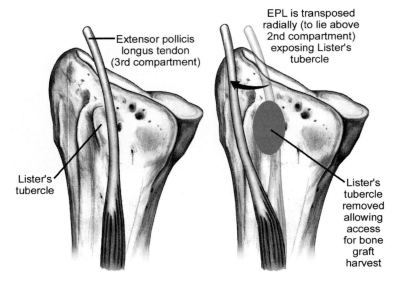

Fig. 3. The extensor pollicis longus (EPL) tendon is transposed radially, aiding exposure (*From* Weiss APC. Principles of limited wrist arthrodesis. In: Berger RA, Weiss APC. Hand surgery. Philadelphia: Lippincott, Williams & Wilkins; 2004. p. 1289–98; with permission.)

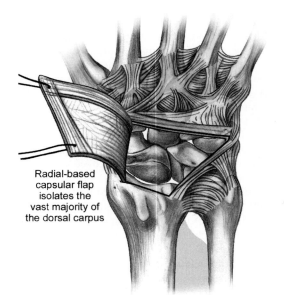

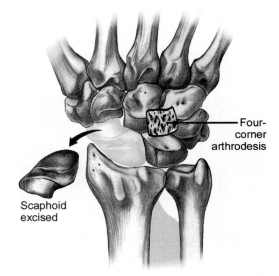

Fig. 4. The ligament-sparing exposure of the carpus. (*From* Weiss APC. Principles of limited wrist arthrodesis. In: Berger RA, Weiss APC. Hand surgery. Philadelphia: Lippincott, Williams & Wilkins; 2004. p. 1289–98; with permission.)

Fig. 5. The scaphoid is excised and used for obtaining some cancellous bone graft. (*From* Weiss APC. Principles of limited wrist arthrodesis. In: Berger RA, Weiss APC. Hand surgery. Philadelphia: Lippincott, Williams & Wilkins; 2004. p. 1289–98; with permission.)

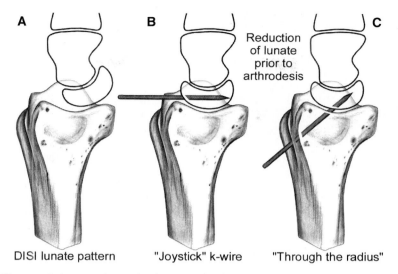

Fig. 6. (*A–C*) Different techniques used to maintain appropriate lunate position during fusion. (*From* Weiss APC. Principles of limited wrist arthrodesis. In: Berger RA, Weiss APC. Hand surgery. Philadelphia: Lippincott, Williams & Wilkins; 2004. p. 1289–98; with permission.)

interstices are packed with autogenous cancellous graft from Lister tubercle or the excised scaphoid.

The eight-hole Spider plate is introduced into the rasped bone. Two screw holes should overlie each carpal bone. While maintaining this plate position, a 1.5-mm drill bit is used to place one self-tapping 2.4-mm cancellous screw in each bone (Fig. 9). The four remaining holes then are drilled and secured with screws of appropriate length. Tightening of all eight screws yields radial compression of the four carpal bones (Fig. 10A,B). The provisional Kirschner wires are removed, and the wrist is brought through a passive range of motion to assure fusion stability and to assess

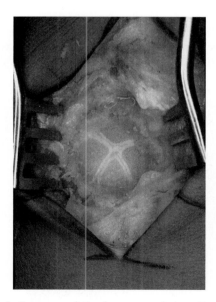

Fig. 7. Exposure of the four-corner fusion site after rasping but before denuding the joint surfaces of cartilage (Courtesy of Arnold-Peter C. Weiss, MD.)

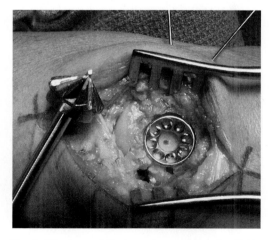

Fig. 8. Check carefully to make sure that the Spider plate is not prominent after rasping to avoid issues of dorsal impingement. (Courtesy of Arnold-Peter C. Weiss, MD.)

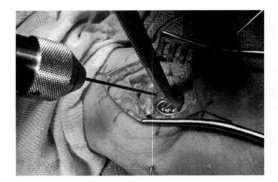

Fig. 9. A special drill guide is used to place screws into the four bones being fused. (Courtesy of Arnold-Peter C. Weiss, MD.)

for dorsal impingement between the plate and distal radius. Intraoperative radiographs are obtained to confirm screw length and carpal alignment (Fig. 11A,B). Particular attention should be directed to the placement of the triquetral screws; avoid screw projection into the pisotriquetral joint. Before closure, the center of the plate and arthrodesis site is packed with any remaining cancellous bone graft.

The wound is irrigated, and the capsule and retinaculum are repaired with 4-0 absorbable sutures. Following skin closure, a short arm splint is applied, allowing for early active range of motion of the fingers and elbow.

Postoperative care and rehabilitation

Watson's four-corner fusion technique implements a long-arm posterior splint for 1 week,

followed by a long-arm intrinsic-plus cast including the thumb, index, and middle fingers. After the fourth week, a short-arm intrinsic-plus cast is maintained for 2 weeks. If the fusion mass seems well healed after 6 weeks, the Kirschner wires are removed and active range of motion is initiated [27].

With Spider plate fixation, sutures are removed after 1 week, and a removable splint or short-arm cast is applied for 3–4 weeks. Early thumb, finger, and elbow range of motion is encouraged. Strenuous activity is prohibited until radiographs confirm bony fusion.

In a 44-month follow-up of 100 patients who had SLAC wrist treated with four-corner fusion, Ashmead and colleagues reported an average flexion/extension arc of 74° (32° extension plus 42° flexion, which was 53% of the uninjured wrist) [13]. Grip strength was 80% compared with the contralateral wrist. Seventy-eight of 85 patients (91%) were satisfied with the result and would undergo the operation again; 61 of 76 patients returned to their original jobs (including all four bilateral patients). A nonunion rate of 3% was reported by the investigator; all nonunions healed after revision bone grafting. Dorsal radiocarpal impingement (resulting from inadequate reduction of the capitolunate joint [32]) was the most frequent late complication, occurring in 13% of patients. After a limited resection of the dorsal distal radius and the abutting dorsal capitate, the patients gained an average of 10% of extension and substantial pain relief.

Cohen and Kozin found that the average wrist range of motion after four-corner fusion was 49° of extension and 31° of flexion, or a 58% flexion–

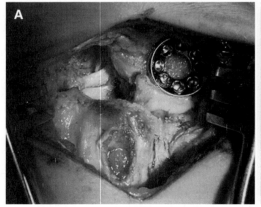
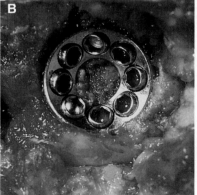

Fig. 10. (A) The Spider plate affixed at the fusion site. (B) A close-up view of the plate's fixation of all four bones. (Courtesy of Arnold-Peter C. Weiss, MD.)

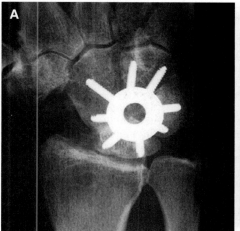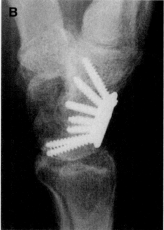

Fig. 11. (*A*) Posteroanterior and (*B*) lateral radiographs demonstrate excellent plate and screw alignment (Courtesy of Arnold-Peter C. Weiss, MD.)

extension arc compared with the contralateral wrist [30]. Grip strength was 79% of the opposite side. The investigators also reported a greater preservation of radioulnar deviation after four-corner fusion versus PRC.

Watson and Ryu followed 20 wrists for an average follow-up of 3 years (range, 16 months to 10.5 years) after undergoing four-corner fusion for SLAC arthritis. The patients averaged 60% of flexion–extension and radioulnar deviation compared with the uninjured wrist. One nonunion was reported (5%) and no patient changed vocation as a result of the fusion [33].

In reviewing the intercarpal arthrodesis literature between 1924 and 1994, Siegel and Ruby reported a four-corner fusion nonunion rate of 4.3% [34]. This was the lowest rate of all intercarpal fusions. In a similar review of the literature between 1946 and 1993, Larsen and colleagues reported a four-corner nonunion range of 9% (Krakauer) to 50% (McAuliffe), and an overall average of 8.4% [35].

Shin's review of eight series and a total of 431 four-corner fusions shed light on the procedure's most common complications. Dorsal radiocarpal impingement was the complication reported most commonly (4.4%) [31], followed by reflex sympathetic dystrophy (3%), and superficial infection (3%). Deep infection occurred in 0.5% and the failure rate (requiring revision to a total wrist arthrodesis) was 2%. The complication rate was 13.5% overall.

Summary

The scaphoid plays a critical role in maintaining normal carpal kinematics. SLAC and SNAC wrist arthritis demonstrate the ramifications of scaphoid pathology on wrist biomechanics. In the past, symptomatic SLAC or SNAC pathology spelled total wrist arthrodesis. Over the past 20 years there has been a movement toward limited wrist arthrodesis in the treatment of SLAC/SNAC wrists. In the long-term follow-up of four-corner fusions, patient satisfaction is high, patients are able to return to their previous vocation, and wrist function averages 60%–70% of the contralateral wrist. The Spider plate is a recent advancement in the four-corner fusion armamentarium that has thus far shown great promise in respect to fusion rates (100% in the first documented series [36]), functional range of motion, intercarpal stability [37], and patient satisfaction.

References

[1] Weber ER. Biomechanical implications of scaphoid waist fractures. Clin Orthop 1980;149:83.

[2] Tomaino MM, Miller RJ, Burton RI. Outcome assessment following limited wrist fusion: objective wrist scoring vx. Patient satisfaction. Contemp Orthop 1994;28:403–10.

[3] Fisk GR. Carpal instability and fractured scaphoid. Ann R Coll Sur Engl 1970;46:63.

[4] Linscheid RL, Dobyns JH, Beabout JW, et al. Traumatic instability of the wrist. J Bone Joint Surg [Am] 1972;54:1612–32.

[5] Gelberman RH, Wolock BS, Siegel DB. Fractures and nonunions of the carpal scaphoid. J Bone Joint Surg [Am] 1989;71:1560–5.

[6] Kobayashi M, Berger RA, Linscheid RL, et al. Intercarpal kinematics during wrist motion. Hand Clin 1997;13:143–9.

[7] Gellman H, Kauffman D, Lenihan M, et al. An in vitro analysis of wrist motion: the effect of limited intercarpal arthrodesis and the contributions of the radiocarpal and midcarpal joints. J Hand Surg [Am] 1988;13:378–83.

[8] Garcia-Elias M, Cooney WP, An KN, et al. Wrist kinematics after limited intercarpal arthrodesis. J Hand Surg [Am] 1989;14:791–9.

[9] Garcia-Elias M, Horii E, Berger RA. Individual carpal bone motion. In: An KN, Berger RA, Cooney WP, editors. Biomechanics of the wrist joint. New York: Springer-Verlag; 1991.

[10] Ruby LK, Cooney WP, An KN, et al. Relative motion of selected carpal bones: a kinematic analysis of the normal wrist. J Hand 1988;13A:1–10.

[11] Linscheid RL. Kinematic considerations of the wrist. Clin Orthop 1986;202:27–39.

[12] Harrington RH, Lichtman DM, Brockmole DM. Common pathways of degenerative arthritis of the wrist. Hand Clin 1987;3:507–25.

[13] Ashmead D IV, Watson HK, Damon C, et al. SLAC wrist salvage. J Hand Surg [Am] 1994;19: 741–50.

[14] Mack GR, Bosse MJ, Gelberman RH, et al. The natural history of scaphoid nonunion. J Bone Joint Surg [Am] 1984;66:504–9.

[15] Leslie IJ, Dickson RA. The fractured carpal scaphoid: natural history and factors influencing outcome. J Bone Joint Surg [Br] 1981;63:225–30.

[16] Barr JS, Elliston WA, Musnick H, et al. Fracture of the carpal navicular (scaphoid) bone. J Bone Joint Surg [Am] 1953;35:609.

[17] Monsivais JJ, Nitz PA, Scully TJ. The role of carpal instability in scaphoid nonunion: casual or causal? J Hand Surg [Br] 1986;11:201–6.

[18] Morimoto H, Tada K, Yoshida T, et al. The relationship between the site of nonunion of the scaphoid and scaphoid nonunion advanced collapse (SNAC). J Bone Joint Surg [Br] 1999;81:871–6.

[19] Obrien ET. Acute fractures and dislocations of the carpus. Orthop Clin N Am 1984;15:237.

[20] Russe O. Fracture of the carpal navicular: diagnosis, non-operative treatment, and operative treatment. J Bone Joint Surg [Am] 1960;42:759–68.

[21] Ruby LK, Stinson J, Belsky MR. The natural history of scaphoid nonunion: a review of fifty cases. J Bone Joint Surg [Am] 1985;67:428–32.

[22] Swanson AB, DeGroot-Swanson G, Maupin BK. Flexible implant arthroplasty of the radiocarpal joint: surgical technique and long-term study. Clin Orthop 1984;187:94–106.

[23] Volz RG. Total wrist arthroplasty: a clinical review. Clin Orthop 1984;187:112–20.

[24] Fitzgerald JP, Peimer CA, Smith RJ. Distraction resection arthroplasty of the wrist. J Hand Surg 1989; 14A:774–81.

[25] Thornton L. Old dislocation of os magnum: open reduction and stabilization. South Med J 1924;17:430.

[26] Krakauer JK, Bishop AT, Cooney WP. Surgical treatment of scapholunate advanced collapse. J Hand Surg [Am] 1994;19:751–9.

[27] Watson HK, Ryu J. Degenerative disorders of the carpus. Orthop Clin N Am 1984;15:337–53.

[28] Berger RA, Bishop AT, Bettinger PC. New dorsal capsulotomy for surgical exposure of the wrist. Ann Plast Surg 1995;35:54–9.

[29] Linscheid RL, Rettig ME. The treatment of displaced scaphoid nonunion with trapezoidal bone graft. In: Gelberman RH, editor. Master techniques in orthopaedic surgery. New York: Raven Press; 1994. p. 119–31.

[30] Cohen MS, Kozin SH. Degenerative arthritis of the wrist: proximal row carpectomy versus scaphoid excision and four-corner arthrodesis. J Hand Surg [Am] 2001;26:94–104.

[31] Shin AY. Four-corner arthrodesis. J Am Soc Surg Hand 2001;1:93–111.

[32] Tomaino MM, Miller RJ, Cole I, et al. Scapholunate advanced collapse wrist: proximal row carpectomy or limited wrist arthrodesis with scaphoid excision. J Hand Surg [Am] 1994;19:134–42.

[33] Watson HK, Ryu J. Evolution of arthritis of the wrist. Clin Orthop 1986;202:57–67.

[34] Siegel JM, Ruby LK. A critical look at intercarpal arthrodesis: a review of the literature. J Hand Surg [Am] 1996;21:717–23.

[35] Larsen CF, Jacoby RA, McCabe SJ. Nonunion rates of limited intercarpal arthrodesis: a meta-analysis of the literature. J Hand Surg [Am] 1997; 22:66–73.

[36] Farvarger N, Jovanovic B, Piaget F, et al. Four corner arthrodesis using the Spider plate [abstract]. Amsterdam: European Federation of Surgical Societies of the Hand; 2002.

[37] Brown RE, Erdmann D. Complications of 50 consecutive limited wrist fusions by a single surgeon. Ann Plast Surg 1995;35:46–53.

ELSEVIER
SAUNDERS

Hand Clin 21 (2005) 539–543

HAND
CLINICS

Scaphotrapeziotrapezoid Arthrodesis for Arthritis

Ronit Wollstein, MD[a,b,c,d], H. Kirk Watson, MD[e,f,g],*

[a]Department of Surgery, Division of Plastic and Reconstructive Surgery, University of Pittsburgh
Medical Center, 200 Lothrop Street, Pittsburgh, PA 15213-2582, USA
[b]University of Pittsburgh Medical Center, Presbyterian Hospital, 200 Lothrop Street,
Pittsburgh, PA 15213-2582, USA
[c]University of Pittsburgh Medical Center, Southside Hospital, 2000 Mary Street, Pittsburgh, PA 15203
[d]Hand Service, VA Hospital of Pittsburgh, Pittsburgh, PA, USA
[e]Department of Orthopaedic Surgery, University of Connecticut School of Medicine,
263 Farmington Avenue, Farmington, CT 06030, USA
[f]Department of Surgery, Yale School of Medicine, 333 Cedar Street, New Haven, CT 06520-8041, USA
[g]Connecticut Combined Hand Surgery Fellowship, 85 Seymore Street, #816, Hartford, CT 06106, USA

Scaphotrapeziotrapezoid arthrodesis (STT) fusion has been used as treatment and prevention for various types of arthritis in the wrist. The main indications in the literature have been for isolated STT arthritis, rotary subluxation of the scaphoid, and Kienbock disease.

Most investigators [1–3] believe there is a spectrum of injury to the wrist leading to a predictable pattern of arthritis. Twenty-five percent of normal asymptomatic adults can be shown to have scapholunate tears of some degree [4]. If the scaphoid proximal pole can displace sufficiently from beneath the capitate, the wrist is subject to what has been described as scapholunate advanced collapse (SLAC) wrist [5] degeneration and a similar pattern that manifests in scaphoid nonunion. This first entails destruction of the radioscaphoid joint, specifically at the radial styloid, and then the rest of this joint. With time and use, arthritis develops between the lunate and capitate and occasionally the lunate and hamate. The radiolunate joint usually is spared in perpetuity [6]. STT fusion is indicated in the treatment of rotary subluxation of the scaphoid before the appearance of degenerative changes (Fig. 1). In Kienbock disease, STT fusion

has been used to "unload" the lunate and provide a usable power transfer across the wrist.

Arthritis in the wrist also can appear in any isolated joint in the wrist. Isolated STT arthritis has a reported incidence of up to 83.3% in cadavers. This can be a consequence of direct trauma to the joint, though this is rare [7–9]. Clinical isolated STT joint arthritis is rare, approximately 10%. The reason for the high percentage of arthritis in this joint in cadavers is unclear. Periscaphoid ligament damage may allow the distal scaphoid to displace radially out from under the trapezium and trapezoid. Then the cartilage of this STT joint is shear loaded, and degenerative arthritis occurs at the STT joint instead of at the radius–scaphoid joint. People tend to live with synovitis at the STT joint and arthritis can be an incidental finding in elderly patients who have minimal symptoms. The anatomy of this joint predilects degenerative change, but the joint displaces easily under load unlike the radioscaphoid or capitate lunate joints. This unloading allows for symptomatic tolerance in the presence of degenerative arthritis.

STT arthritis also can accompany basal joint thumb arthritis, which is referred to as pan trapezial or the basal joint pain syndrome by Melone [10].

The mainstay of operative treatment in isolated symptomatic STT arthritis is STT fusion [8,11–13]. Other operative options described in the literature include excision of the distal pole

---

* Corresponding author.

E-mail address: hkwatson01@aol.com
(H.K. Watson).

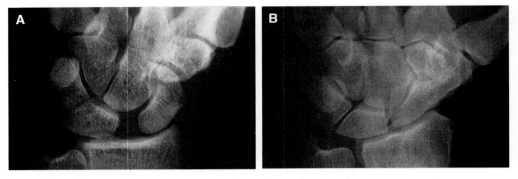

Fig. 1. (*A*, *B*) STT arthrodesis for rotary subluxation of the scaphoid pre- and postoperation.

of the scaphoid [14,15] and arthroscopic debridement [16]. These are partial ablative procedures with possible loss of wrist power from an unloadable scaphoid. This concern has not yet been addressed by long-term follow-up in the literature.

In the authors' series of STT fusions [17], average range of flexion/extension following surgery was 70%–80% of the nonoperated side. Mean grip strength was 77% of the nonoperated side. There was an overall nonunion rate of 4%, but for the degenerative arthritis group (98 patients) the nonunion rate was 2%. The rotational subluxation of the scaphoid (RSS) group had a nonunion rate of 5%. The STT arthritis group was significantly older than the RSS group (median, 54 years of age in the degenerative group as opposed to median 36 years in the RSS group).

The use of STT fusion in the treatment of rotary subluxation of the scaphoid or scapholunate instability has been the subject of much controversy. Notorious for having a high nonunion rate and a high incidence of general complications, this operation has its distractors [18–21]. There is also concern over the ability of this procedure to prevent the appearance of arthritis in rotary subluxation of the scaphoid and the development of arthritis in neighboring joints, most notably SLAC wrist, following fusion of this joint. Abnormally overloading other joints is always a concern when fusing one joint that is part of a movement sequence. Although this long-term sequel has not been ruled out completely, there have been many reports now of good long-term results [17,22–24]. In a review of the literature there have not been any studies substantiating the development of arthritis following STT fusion.

A long-term phenomenon that did arise was impingement developing with the radial styloid following fusion. The authors believe this is an impingement of the scaphoid that can no longer rotate into flexion on the styloid.

Watson and colleagues modified the procedure to include a radial styloidectomy in 1990 [25]. Should this be considered arthritis following the change in the mechanics of the wrist? The answer is not clear, though as already stated, this procedure has not been shown to progress to SLAC wrist.

Alternative techniques for chronic scapholunate instability or RSS are many and have mixed results [26–30]. This remains a fairly common situation with no one good solution. Most techniques attempt to reconstruct the dorsal scapholunate ligament [31–35].

Kienbock disease remains an enigma as to etiology and therefore treatment. The natural history of Kienbock disease also remains unclear [36], making it even more difficult to interpret the results of treatment [37–39]. The different treatment options that have been described have yielded similar results [37,40–47]. In the authors' study, the group of patients who had Kienbock disease had significantly less range of motion following STT fusion when compared with other diagnoses [17]. Recently Meier et al studied the results of 59 patients who had Kienbock disease treated with STT fusion [48]. They found improvement in pain, grip strength, and range of motion. Their postoperative values were 81% of preoperative range of motion and 60% of the normal side, which is consistent with the authors' series (Fig. 2).

Trumble found similar results when comparing different treatment modalities [49]. He also showed that biomechanically, STT fusion and radial shortening were successful in unloading the lunate.

The surgical technique for STT arthrodesis has been described extensively [50]. The authors believe, however, that some technical details are critical to a good outcome.

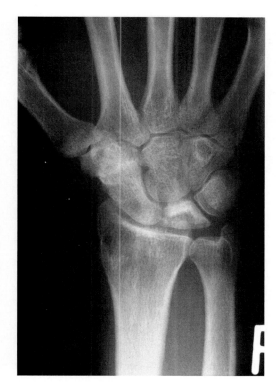

Fig. 2. STT arthrodesis for Kienbock disease.

1. The articular surfaces must be thoroughly de-nuded of cartilage and cortex down to good cancellous bone.
2. The original external dimensions of the STT joint should be maintained by using a spacer when presetting the pins (if pins are used) and carefully packing in a large amount of cancellous bone graft.
3. The scaphoid should lie at an angle of 55°–60° of palmar flexion relative to the long axis of the radius when seen on the lateral view of the wrist.
4. A radial styloidectomy should be performed as part of the operation, taking care not to injure the origin of the volar ligaments.
5. The postoperative protocol should be ad-hered to as stringently as possible, includ-ing 6 weeks in a cast, 3 weeks in a long arm cast that includes the thumb and metacarpo-phalangeal joints in flexion, and then change to a short arm cast, still including the thumb but leaving the fingers free. Smokers rou-tinely are immobilized for an extra week.

The authors' long-term results of STT arthrod-esis for arthritis have been encouraging. A good range of motion together with good strength and function can be achieved [18]. Achieving union, however, can be a challenge and requires strict ad-herence to surgical and postsurgical guidelines. There is a modification for smokers. Also, a surgical procedure that results in any loss of wrist motion is not the ideal solution. It is clear, therefore, why there are endless attempts in the literature and in practice to solve the problem of scapholunate in-stability in other ways. Still, there is a place in the hand surgeons' armamentarium for STT arthrode-sis, certainly for cases of isolated STT arthritis and probably in specific cases with other diagnoses also.

References

[1] Linscheid RL, Dobyns JH, Beckenbaugh RD, et al. Instability patterns of the wrist. J Hand Surg [Am] 1983;8(5 Pt 2):682–6.
[2] Mayfield JK. Mechanism of carpal injuries. Clin Orthop 1980;149:45–54.
[3] Mayfield JK, Johnson RP, Kilcoyne RK. Carpal dislocations: pathomechanics and progressive peri-lunar instability. J Hand Surg [Am] 1980;5(3): 226–41.
[4] Watson HK, Ohoni L, Pitts EC, et al. Rotary sub-luxation of the scaphoid: A spectrum of instability. J Hand Surg [Br] 1993;18:62–4.
[5] Watson HK, Ballet FL. The SLAC wrist: scapholu-nate advanced collapse pattern of degenerative ar-thritis. J Hand Surg [Am] 1984;9(3):358–65.
[6] Vender MI, Watson HK, Wiener BD, et al. Degener-ative change in symptomatic scaphoid nonunion. J Hand Surg [Am] 1987;12(4):514–9.
[7] Chantelot C, Peltier B, Demondion X, et al. A trans STT, trans capitate perilunate dislocation of the car-pus. A case report. Ann Chir Main Memb Super 1999;18(1):61–5.
[8] Wilhelm K, Rolle A, Hild A. The scaphoid-trape-zium-trapezoid arthrosis. A clinical study 1982–1985. Unfallchirurg 1989;92(2):59–63.
[9] Meier R, Prommersberger KJ, Krimmer H. Scapho-trapezio-trapezoid arthrodesis (triscaphe arthrode-sis). Handchir Mikrochir Plast Chir 2003;35(5): 323–7.
[10] Melone CP Jr, Beavers B, Isani A. The basal joint pain syndrome. Clin Orthop 1987;220:58–67.
[11] Viegas SF, Patterson RM, Peterson PD, et al. Evaluation of the biomechanical efficacy of limited intercarpal fusions for the treatment of scapho-lu-nate dissociation. J Hand Surg [Am] 1990;15(1): 120–8.
[12] Watson HK, Ryu J, DiBella A. An approach to Kienbock's disease: triscaphe arthrodesis. J Hand Surg [Am] 1985;10(2):179–87.

[13] Srinivasan VB, Matthews JP. Results of scaphotra-peziotrapezoid fusion for isolated idiopathic arthritis. J Hand Surg [Br] 1996;21(3):378–80.

[14] Garcia-Elias M, Lluch A. Partial excision of scaphoid: is it ever indicated? Hand Clin 2001;17(4): 687–95 [x.].

[15] Hulsbergen-Kruger S, Partecke B. Intercarpal and radiocarpal resection arthroplasty and arthrodesis. Orthopade 1999;28(10):899–906.

[16] Ashwood N, Bain GI, Fogg Q. Results of arthroscopic debridement for isolated scaphotrapeziotrapezoid arthritis. J Hand Surg [Am] 2003;28(5): 729–32.

[17] Watson HK, Wollstein R, Joseph E, et al. Scaphotrapeziotrapezoid arthrodesis: a follow-up study. J Hand Surg [Am] 2003;28(3):397–404.

[18] Kleinman WB, Carroll CT. Scapho-trapezio-trapezoid arthrodesis for treatment of chronic static and dynamic scapho-lunate instability: a 10-year perspective on pitfalls and complications. J Hand Surg [Am] 1990;15(3):408–14.

[19] Kleinman WB. Long-term study of chronic scapholunate instability treated by scapho-trapezio-trapezoid arthrodesis. J Hand Surg [Am] 1989;14(3): 429–45.

[20] Ishida O, Tsai TM. Complications and results of scapho-trapezio-trapezoid arthrodesis. Clin Orthop 1993;287:125–30.

[21] Frykman EB, Af Ekenstam F, Wadin K. Triscaphoid arthrodesis and its complications. J Hand Surg [Am] 1988;13(6):844–9.

[22] Minami A, Kato H, Iwasaki N, et al. Limited wrist fusions: comparison of results 22 and 89 months after surgery. J Hand Surg [Am] 1999;24(1):133–7.

[23] Minami A, Ogino T, Minami M. Limited wrist fusions. J Hand Surg [Am] 1988;13(5):660–7.

[24] Fortin PT, Louis DS. Long-term follow-up of scaphoid-trapezium-trapezoid arthrodesis. J Hand Surg [Am] 1993;18(4):675–81.

[25] Rogers WD, Watson HK. Degenerative arthritis at the triscaphe joint. J Hand Surg [Am] 1990;15(2): 232–5.

[26] Zubairy AI, Jones WA. Scapholunate fusion in chronic symptomatic scapholunate instability. J Hand Surg [Br] 2003;28(4):311–4.

[27] Muermans S, De Smet L, Van Ransbeeck H. Blatt dorsal capsulodesis for scapholunate instability. Acta Orthop Belg 1999;65(4):434–9.

[28] Saffar P, Sokolow C, Duclos L. Soft tissue stabilization in the management of chronic scapholunate instability without osteoarthritis. A 15-year series. Acta Orthop Belg 1999;65(4):424–33.

[29] Uhl RL, Williamson SC, Bowman MW, et al. Dorsal capsulodesis using suture anchors. Am J Orthop 1997;26(8):547–8.

[30] Wintman BI, Gelberman RH, Katz JN. Dynamic scapholunate instability: results of operative treatment with dorsal capsulodesis. J Hand Surg [Am] 1995;20(6):971–9.

[31] Augsburger S, Necking L, Horton J, et al. A comparison of scaphoid-trapezium-trapezoid fusion and four-bone tendon weave for scapholunate dissociation. J Hand Surg [Am] 1992;17(2): 360–9.

[32] Conyers DJ. Scapholunate interosseous reconstruction and imbrication of palmar ligaments. J Hand Surg [Am] 1990;15(5):690–700.

[33] Lutz M, Kralinger F, Goldhahn J, et al. Dorsal scapholunate ligament reconstruction using a periosteal flap of the iliac crest. Arch Orthop Trauma Surg 2004;124(3):197–202.

[34] Minami A, Kato H, Iwasaki N. Treatment of scapholunate dissociation: ligamentous repair associated with modified dorsal capsulodesis. Hand Surg 2003;8(1):1–6.

[35] Wolf JM, Weiss AP. Bone-retinaculum-bone reconstruction of scapholunate ligament injuries. Orthop Clin North Am 2001;32(2):241–6 [viii.].

[36] Watson HK, Guidera PM. Aetiology of Kienbock's Disease. J Hand Surg [Br] 1997;22(1):5–7.

[37] Keith PP, Nuttall D, Trail I. Long-term outcome of nonsurgically managed Kienbock's disease. J Hand Surg [Am] 2004;29(1):63–7.

[38] Taniguchi Y, Nakao S, Tamaki T. Incidentally diagnosed Kienbock's disease. Clin Orthop 2002;395: 121–7.

[39] Beckenbaugh RD, Shives TC, Dobyns JH, et al. Kienbock's disease: the natural history of Kienbock's disease and consideration of lunate fractures. Clin Orthop 1980;149:98–106.

[40] Kato H, Usui M, Minami A. Long-term results of Kienbock's disease treated by excisional arthroplasty with a silicone implant or coiled palmaris longus tendon. J Hand Surg [Am] 1986;11(5): 645–53.

[41] Kristensen SS, Thomassen E, Christensen F. Kienbock's disease—late results by non-surgical treatment. A follow-up study. J Hand Surg [Br] 1986; 11(3):422–5.

[42] Nakamura R, Imaeda T, Miura T. Radial shortening for Kienbock's disease: factors affecting the operative result. J Hand Surg [Br] 1990; 15(1):40–5.

[43] Kuhlmann JN, Kron C, Boabighi A, et al. Vascularised pisiform bone graft. Indications, technique and long-term results. Acta Orthop Belg 2003;69(4): 311–6.

[44] Strackee SD. Wedge osteotomies of the radius for Kienbock's disease. J Hand Surg [Am] 2002;27(5): 917; author reply, 8.

[45] Shin AY, Bishop AT. Pedicled vascularized bone grafts for disorders of the carpus: scaphoid nonunion and Kienbock's disease. J Am Acad Orthop Surg 2002;10(3):210–6.

[46] Wada A, Miura H, Kubota H, et al. Radial closing wedge osteotomy for Kienbock's disease: an over 10 year clinical and radiographic follow-up. J Hand Surg [Br] 2002;27(2):175–9.

[47] Soejima O, Iida H, Komine S, et al. Lateral closing wedge osteotomy of the distal radius for advanced stages of Kienbock's disease. J Hand Surg [Am] 2002;27(1):31–6.

[48] Meier R, van Griensven M, Krimmer H. Scaphotrapeziotrapezoid (STT)-arthrodesis in Kienbock's disease. J Hand Surg [Br] 2004;29(6):580–4.

[49] Trumble T, Glisson RR, Seaber AV, et al. A biomechanical comparison of the methods for treating Kienbock's disease. J Hand Surg [Am] 1986;11(1):88–93.

[50] Watson HK, Weinzweig J. Triscaphe arthrodesis. In: Watson HK, Weinzweig J, editors. The wrist. Philadelphia: Lippincott, Williams and Wilkins; 2001. p. 931–8.

ELSEVIER
SAUNDERS

Hand Clin 21 (2005) 545–552

HAND
CLINICS

Partial Arthrodesis for the Rheumatoid Wrist

Daniel B. Herren, MD[a],*, Hajime Ishikawa, MD[b]

[a]Handsurgery Department, Schulthess Klinik, Lengghalde 2, 8008, Zurich, Switzerland
[b]Rheumatic Center, Niigata Prefectural Senami Hospital,
Senami Onsen 2-4-15 Murakami, Niigata, 958-0037 Japan

Patterns of wrist deformity

The wrist is one of the main targets of rheumatoid arthritis [1] and may deteriorate rapidly despite current modern medical management. With a cumulative incidence of wrist involvement of more than 70% 3 years after the onset of disease and of 95% after 11 years, wrist treatment is the key to preserving hand function.

The classic pattern of deformity and destruction shows involvement of the radiocarpal and the radioulnar joint with destabilization of the carpus caused by attenuation of the extrinsic wrist ligaments [2], resulting in an ulnar–palmar translocation and supination of the wrist [3–6]. Three main pathophysiologic factors play the most important role in the process of wrist deformation: cartilage destruction, synovial expansion, and ligamentous laxity. The cartilage thinning is caused by cytochemical effects with continuous degradation [7,8]. Bony erosion is caused by the synovial expansion, particularly at the site of vascular penetration into the bone, such as the radial origin of the Testut ligament. This causes stretching of the retaining intrinsic and extrinsic wrist ligaments with deformation [3,9]. One of the most important intrinsic structures, the scapholunate interval starts to dissociate and continues to disintegrate the internal architecture of the carpus. The force vector across the wrist predominately acts in a palmar–ulnar direction. With ongoing destruction of the wrist, these muscles lose their physiologic moment arms and become a deforming force [3,10].

Natural course of the rheumatoid wrist

Although considered a uniform disease of immunogenetic background [7], patients show various courses of the disease, especially at the wrist level. Ten to 20 years after wrist involvement, progressive radiologic deterioration settles down into a stable or unstable form [11,12]. Because functional loss is obviously greater for the unstable forms with tendon imbalance and loss of power [13], the recognition of the pattern of progression may have implications on management and surgical treatment. The identification of an unstable form in the early stage of the disease and the conversion into a stable form is an important concept for preserving wrist and hand function over time [11,14–24].

Most currently used classifications of the wrist deformity in rheumatoid arthritis highlight the actual destruction of the carpus and do not include the different possible patterns of progression [25–27]. Stanley and colleagues tried to incorporate more practical guidelines in their rheumatoid wrist classification schemes [26,28–30]. Both classifications, however, still lack the ability to anticipate future development of wrist destruction. Based on radiologic long-term analysis. Simmen [12] and Flury [11] proposed a new classification of rheumatoid wrist involvement considering the type of destruction in relation to the possible future development of the disease with direct consequences for surgical decisions. Three patterns of wrist involvement are distinguished based on the morphology of destruction over the course of the disease. Serial radiographs are needed to classify the wrists into type I, II, or III. Type I rheumatoid wrists show a spontaneous tendency for ankylosis (Fig. 1), type II wrists show a destruction pattern

---

* Corresponding author.
E-mail address: hed@kws.ch (D.B. Herren).

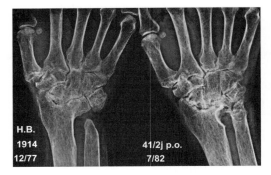

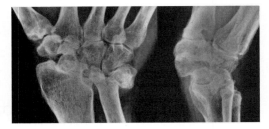

Fig. 3. Type IIIa wrist with an unstable ligamentous support and deformation with complete carpal collapse and extreme ulnar drift.

Fig. 1. Type I wrist with a tendency of spontaneous fusion of the midcarpal and radiocarpal joint.

similar to osteoarthritic wrists with a relative stability over time (Fig. 2), and type III wrists show a disintegration with progressive destruction and loss of alignment. Type III wrist, by definition unstable forms of deformation, are further subdivided into type IIIa (Fig. 3) with more ligamentous instability and type IIIb (Fig. 4) with marked destruction of the bone resulting in a complete loss of the carpal architecture.

The classification is based on serial radiographs taken in an interval between 6 and 12 months, with measurement of carpal height ratio and ulnar translation. Borisch and colleagues [31] recommend the use of the measurement method described by Boumann 1994 [32] with a higher applicability and sensitivity compared with the Chamay index and the Youm index. Flury could show that a change in the carpal height ratio of more than 0.015 or the increase of ulnar translation of more than 1.5 mm per year classifies a wrist into the unstable type III category. With these criteria it is possible that most wrists can be classified,

although in some cases of type II involvement a shift from stable to unstable during the disease could be observed. Zangger and colleagues [14] investigated the liability of this classification system in patients who had early rheumatoid arthritis. The intraobserver agreement was good and there was consistency over time. In only approximately 50% of patients who had early disease, however, could the classification be applied.

In the rheumatoid wrist the destruction of the various compartments differs from the destruction observed in degenerative or traumatic SLAC-wrist patterns. Although in the SLAC situation the radioscaphoid joint suffers the most, followed by the midcarpal joint, in the patient who has rheumatoid arthritis the radiolunate joint deteriorates first, before the radioscaphoid facet. The midcarpal joint is preserved for longer. Anatomically the radiocarpal joint is less stable than the midcarpal joint and is subject to greater destruction caused by the instability of the disease process [33].

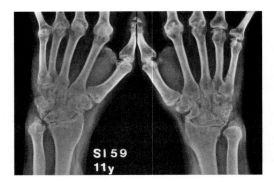

Fig. 2. Type II wrist representing a more arthritic-arthritis type of destruction with preservation of the bone stock and no gross destabilization radiocarpal.

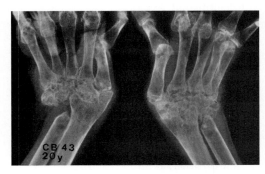

Fig. 4. Type IIIb wrist with complete loss of the bony architecture.

Wrist synovectomy and distal ulna resection

The first attempt to standardize a surgical procedure to treat the rheumatoid wrist was introduced by Backdahl [34]. He described the term "caput ulnae syndrome" and recommended the surgical resection of the ulnar head together with a synovectomy of the wrist extensor tendons to prevent tendon rupture. This concept worked for a significant number of patients; however, there was the observation that over time the carpal collapse continued. Thirupathi and colleagues [35] observed 7 years after dorsal wrist synovectomy and distal ulna resection good pain relief, stable tendon conditions, and a preserved functional range of motion. Carpal collapse and translocation could not be predicted by preoperative radiographs, however, and progression of carpal dislocation continued in a linear fashion with the time of follow-up. Similar results were found by Masada and colleagues [36], and they recommended distal ulnar resection only in patients who have a stable wrist configuration. Ishikawa found in 43 patients treated with a distal ulnar resection, wrist and extensor synovectomy, in the long term, a significant acceleration of ulnar translation in treated versus untreated wrists was observed, whereas the carpal collapse and the palmar subluxation progressed parallel to the untreated opposite wrist [37]. These investigators therefore recommended some stabilizing procedure to prevent ulnar carpal shift.

A Sauve-Kapandji procedure

1985 Alnot and colleagues [27] recommended for further wrist stabilization the preservation of the distal radioulnar joint with a Sauve-Kapandji procedure. Their retrospective follow-up study proved after 2.5 years a clinical and radiologic stabilizing effect of this procedure. Chantelot and colleagues [38] basically confirmed theses results but also found an increased ulnar shift and radial deviation postoperatively over time. They suggested a tendon transfer of the extensor carpi radialis longus tendon to the extensor carpi radialis brevis to prevent further radial deviation.

Indications: radiolunate/radioscapholunate/ radiolunotriquetral arthrodesis

Stack and Vaughan-Jackson [39] in 1971 were the first who reported about a patient who had rheumatoid arthritis in whom ulnar drift of the fingers was prevented by spontaneous radiolunate fusion. Chamay [40] found in his series in 13% of the rheumatoid wrists a spontaneous radiolunate fusion with longstanding stability and still functional mobility. He applied this observation to the treatment of rheumatoid deformities in unstable wrist situations in which the midcarpal joint space was preserved. The idea of radiolunate partial arthrodesis includes the realignment of the subluxed carpus by reduction of the proximal carpal row. It is still unclear, however, if the reduction in the radiolunate fusion should be as physiologic as possible. Borisch and colleagues [41] found a significant ongoing destruction of the midcarpal joint after radiolunate fusion, especially in cases with fixed carpal collapse preoperatively. The reposition of these wrists caused a midcarpal dislocation or rotation, which causes secondary destruction of the midcarpal joint. They recommend in these cases the fixation of the lunate in the existing anatomic location.

In patients who have advanced destruction of the radiocarpal joint, the partial fusion may be expanded to a radioscapholunate (RSL) arthrodesis [42]. Taleisnik [33] went one step further and proposed an RSL fusion combined with a midcarpal arthroplasty consisting of a silicone implant. There were no further publications about this treatment. There are no larger series with results of pure RSL fusions in rheumatoid arthritis.

In cases of advanced destruction of the lunate and difficult bone situations, the radiolunate arthrodesis may be performed by inclusion of the triquetrum to the fusion site (radiolunotriquetral [RLT]). This facilitates the use of hardware and enhances the stability of the construct.

Range of motion

An overall review of the literature shows good clinical results with high patient satisfaction for limited wrist fusion procedures in patients who have rheumatoid arthritis [29,43–51]. There is a wide variation in the postoperative range of motion in these patients. Doets and colleagues [52] observed a postoperative increase in mobility in all directions with the exception of wrist flexion. Borisch [41] and Schill [53] noted a decrease in the range of motion in all planes, but again, most significantly for wrist flexion. This corresponds to the authors' experience, with a decrease of wrist motion in all directions but only significantly for wrist flexion. The range of motion for pure radiolunate (RL) fusion ranged in a long-term follow-up series from 57°–39° flexion/extension, representing 68% of the preoperative mobility. If the scaphoid was included in the fusion side (RSL fusion), it remained 52% of the preoperative motion with a range from 50°–26° for flexion/extension. The few patients (n = 3) in the same series with an RLT fusion had a preservation rate of 84% of preoperative wrist flexion/extension, but started with less motion and had absolute values from 45°–38°. There are some clinical observations that the range of motion may depend on the integrity of the scapholunate junction. Cases in which the proximal row shifts as a unit, with an intact scapholunate ligament, are stiffer with an RL fusion compared with wrists with a complete disruption of the scapholunate interval.

In summary, it may be expected that two thirds to one half of the preoperative range of motion may be preserved with a partial fusion of the proximal carpal row to the radius in rheumatoid wrists. The main loss observed is in wrist flexion. Forearm pronation and supination increase significantly in most cases because of the resection of the distal ulna.

Radiologic changes

The most interesting aspect of the partial arthrodesis of the rheumatoid wrist is the long-term fate. Besides the stabilizing nature of this intervention, it was speculated that the ongoing destruction could be stopped or at least could decelerate further deterioration. Borisch and colleagues [41] found 5 years after RL fusion a further

arthritic destruction of the midcarpal joint in 37% of cases. Della Santa and Chamay [48] compared 26 operated (RL fusion) and 20 untreated rheumatoid wrists after 5 years. They found ongoing dislocation of the wrist despite the stabilizing procedure. The speed of deterioration depended on the type of wrist involvement and was faster in the disintegration type (Simmen type III). Rittmeister and colleagues [51] compared the results of RL arthrodesis with total wrist fusion (Mannerfelt technique). Wrist pain and swelling were better controlled with a total wrist fusion, whereas grip strength was better in the partial fusion wrists. Carpal degeneration advanced with follow-up time in the patients who had partial fusion. That investigator recommended radiolunate fusion for the nondominant hand in patients who had slow carpal progression of the disease only.

The authors' own long-term results (HI) of RL, RSL, and RLT arthrodesis in rheumatoid arthritis differ slightly from previous publications [50]. After a minimal follow-up of 10 years a durable effect in prevention of ulnar translation and palmar carpal subluxation could be shown (Figs. 5 and 6). Carpal collapse improved initially, however, but returned to the preoperative level after 5 years. The progression of the osteoarthritic changes at the midcarpal level varied. In two thirds of the wrists the midcarpal joint remained fairly well preserved after 10 years. Above all it could be shown that in some of the patients the partial fusion had an impressive protective character for carpal joint destruction in the long term (Fig. 7).

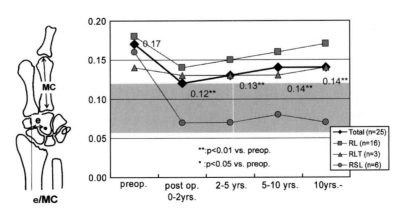

Fig. 5. Measurement of ulnar carpal shift ratio (e/MC). MC, length of the third metacarpal. Changes in the ulnar carpal shift ratio after radiocarpal stabilization. The shaded area indicates the normal range (mean ± SD). RL, radiolunate arthrodesis; RLT, radiolunotriquetral arthrodesis; RSL, radioscapholunate arthrodesis; Total, RL+RLT+RSL.

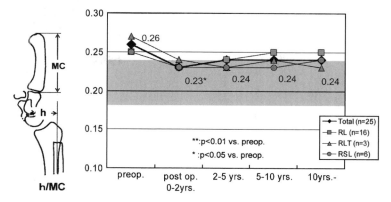

Fig. 6. Measurement of palmar carpal subluxation ratio h/MC. Changes in the palmar carpal subluxation ratio after radiocarpal stabilization. The shaded area indicates the normal range (mean ± SD). RL, radiolunate arthrodesis; RLT, radiolunotriquetral arthrodesis; RSL, radioscapholunate arthrodesis; Total, RL+RLT+RSL.

The pathophysiologic destruction pattern in rheumatoid arthritis solely allows partial arthrodesis, which crosses the radiocarpal joint. All other concepts like midcarpal fusion in all its variations and proximal row carpectomy do not work in the rheumatoid wrist. The ligamentous instability together with the bone destruction always lead the radiocarpal joint to an ulnar/palmar movement.

Alternatives to the RL, RSL, and the RLT arthrodesis remain total wrist arthrodesis or total wrist arthroplasty. It is widely accepted that wrist joints with an aggressive type of the disease, refractory synovitis, a type III wrist according to the Schulthess classification, and severe destruction of the midcarpal joint are contraindications for partial wrist fusion in rheumatoid arthritis. The conversion of a partial arthrodesis to a total

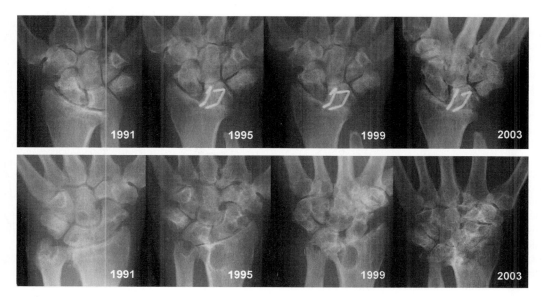

Fig. 7. Serial radiographs over a period of 10 years in the same patient. On the right wrist (upper row) a radiolunate fusion, combined with a synovectomy and a Darrach ulna resection was performed. The carpus was stable over the observation period. The opposite left wrist remained untreated and showed a marked progression of the carpus destruction with ongoing ulnar carpal shift.

wrist fusion is technically without any specific difficulties. In contrast, the preservation of the bone stock in partial fusion facilitates the wrist fusion procedure. The clinical experience shows few cases in which this had to be performed.

Surgical technique

The rheumatoid wrist is approached by way of a dorsal straight incision centered over the axis of the third metacarpal. The skin flaps are well raised over to the radial and the ulnar sensible nerve branches, which must be visualized. The extensor retinaculum is split longitudinally in the interval between the fifth and sixth compartment or at the ulnar border of the sixth compartment. An extensor tenosynovectomy is performed and the terminal branch of the dorsal interosseous nerve is resected as part of a partial wrist denervation procedure. The distal end of the ulna is resected in a length of 1.5–2.0 cm and a synovectomy of the distal radioulnar joint is performed. The wrist joint capsule is incised in the axis of the capitate, and two triangular flaps are raised from the radius. Alternatively, a fiber-splitting approach described by Berger and Bishop [54] can be used. This gives access to the radiocarpal and the midcarpal joints and synovectomy can be performed. The inspection of the radiocarpal joint and the bone destruction pattern then allows the choice of intervention. RL fusion is performed when the radioscaphoid fossa is preserved. If there is further destruction, the RSL fusion option is chosen. In cases of severe deformation of the lunate, an RLT technique may be applied. The remaining cartilage of the surface, which will be fused, is removed to the level of subchondral cancellous bone. If the curvature of both elements is preserved, the reposition and fixation is facilitated. The lunate is repositioned so that the radius covers approximately two thirds of the lunate, which corresponds to its original position. Unlike some investigators, the authors recommend reducing the lunate as physiologically as possible. The reduction is held with K-wires. It may be easier to insert these wires from the triquetrum through the lunate to the radius. Fluoroscopic radiographic examination is mandatory to confirm the correct desired position of the lunate in all planes. The K-wires still allow some distension of the fusion side, and the bone graft, harvested from the resected distal ulna, may be affected. The final internal fixation may be realized with titanium power staples (length × width = 10 mm × 13 mm or 15 mm

× 13 mm) or, when good bone quality is present, with a 2.0-mm minicondylar or T-plate (Fig. 8). The arrangement of the staples is critical. Ideally 2–3 staples should be placed in three-dimensional different converging angles to prevent redislocation. Alternatively a sliding cortical bone graft with two screws may be applied. The RLT arthrodesis is best performed with K-wires that are left percutaneous and later must be removed. The ulnar stump may be stabilized with the pronator quadratus flap, which is wrapped around the ulna and sutured to the dorsal periosteum.

The wrist capsule then is closed and the extensor retinaculum is divided with the distal half being placed under the extensor tendons to reinforce the wrist capsule and to cover the implant. A short arm cast or splint is applied for 6–8 weeks. The first radiographic control after 6 weeks usually shows evidence of healing, and wrist mobilization can be started.

It is possible to combine this wrist procedure with surgery to other locations in the hand. Concomitant small joint fusion or arthroplasty is possible and does not compromise the rehabilitation process. In cases of staged procedures, according to the principal rules of rheumatoid surgery timing, the proximal elements should be addressed first (eg, wrist before metacarpo-phalangeal joints).

Complications

Main complications consist of inappropriate hardware placement and nonunion. Wetzel [24]

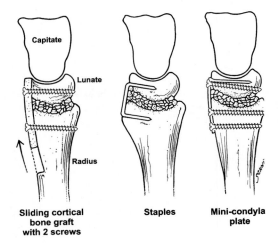

Fig. 8. Different techniques for radiolunate fusion. (*From* Herren DB, Simmen BR. Limited and complete fusion of the rheumatoid wrist. J Am Soc Surg Hand 2002;2:21–32; with permission.)

reported on two broken mini T-plates out of 33 operated patients. Doets and colleagues [50] observed malplacement of staples in the midcarpal joint in one third of the patients in whom no intraoperative radiologic control was performed. Nonunion rates in this type of intervention are low. Redislocation of the radiocarpal joint seems to be of more concern. Stable internal fixation with correct placement of the hardware is crucial. Patients suffering from an aggressive type of destruction may show further deterioration of the carpus; in some of them the lunate may remain in place while the rest of the carpus might melt around the stable element. The determination of the type of destruction is important and indications for surgical treatment must be chosen carefully.

References

[1] Hamalainen M, Kammonen M, Lehtimaki M. Epidemiology of wrist involvement in rheumatoid arthritis. Rheumatology 1992;17(1–7):1–7.

[2] Taleisnik J. Rheumatoid arthritis at the wrist. Hand Clin 1989;5(2):257–78.

[3] Shapiro JS. The wrist in rheumatoid arthritis. Hand Clin 1996;12(3):477–98.

[4] Pahle JA, Raunio P. The influence of wrist position on finger deviation in the rheumatoid hand. A clinical and radiological study. J Bone Joint Surg [Br] 1969;51(4):664–76.

[5] Straub LR, Ranawat CS. The wrist in rheumatoid arthritis. Surgical treatment and results. J Bone Joint Surg [Am] 1969;51(1):1–20.

[6] Hastings DE, Evans JA. Rheumatoid wrist deformities and their relation to ulnar drift. J Bone Joint Surg [Am] 1975;57(7):930–4.

[7] Harris ED Jr. Rheumatoid arthritis. Pathophysiology and implications for therapy. N Engl J Med 1990;322(18):1277–89.

[8] Cush J, Lipsky P. Cellular basis of rheumatoid inflammation. Clin Orthop 1991;265:9–22.

[9] Ritt M, Stuart P, Berglund L, et al. Rotational stability of the carpus relative to the forearm. J Hand Surg 1995;20:305–11.

[10] Shapiro JS. A new factor in the etiology of ulnar drift. Clin Orthop 1970;68:32–43.

[11] Flury MP, Herren DB, Simmen BR. Rheumatoid arthritis of the wrist. Classification related to the natural course. Clin Orthop 1999;366:72–7.

[12] Simmen BR, Huber H. The wrist joint in chronic polyarthritis—a new classification based on the type of destruction in relation to the natural course and the consequences for surgical therapy. Handchir Mikrochir Plast Chir 1994;26(4):182–9.

[13] Clayton ML. Surgical treatment at the wrist in rheumatoid arthritis: a review of thirty-seven patients. J Bone Joint Surg [Am] 1965;47:741–50.

[14] Zangger P, Kachura J, Bogoch E. The Simmen classification of wrist destruction in rheumatoid arthritis. Experience in patients with early disease. J Hand Surg [Br] 1999;24(4):400–4.

[15] Mannerfelt L. Surgical treatment of the rheumatoid wrist and aspects of the natural course when untreated. Clin Rheum Dis 1984;10(3):549–70.

[16] Kobus RJ, Turner RH. Wrist arthrodesis for treatment of rheumatoid arthritis. J Hand Surg [Am] 1990;15(4):541–6.

[17] Linscheid RL. Surgery for rheumatoid arthritis—timing and techniques: the upper extremity. J Bone Joint Surg [Am] 1968;50(3):605–13.

[18] Allieu Y, Brahin B, Asencio G, et al. The surgical treatment of the rheumatoid wrist. Current perspectives. Ann Chir Main 1984;3(1):58–65.

[19] Carroll RE, Dick HM. Arthrodesis of the wrist for rheumatoid arthritis. J Bone Joint Surg [Am] 1971;53(7):1365–9.

[20] Murphy DM, Khoury JG, Imbriglia JE, et al. Comparison of arthroplasty and arthrodesis for the rheumatoid wrist. J Hand Surg [Am] 2003;28(4):570–6.

[21] O'Brien ET. Surgical principles and planning for the rheumatoid hand and wrist. Clin Plast Surg 1996;23(3):407–20.

[22] Vahvanen V, Kettunen P. Arthrodesis of the wrist in rheumatoid arthritis. A follow-up study of 62 cases. Ann Chir Gynaecol 1977;66(4):195–202.

[23] Vainio K. Surgery of rheumatoid arthritis. Surg Ann 1974;6:309–35.

[24] Wetzel R, Wessinghage D. Arthrodesis of the wrist joint in patients with polyarthritis. Handchir Mikrochir Plast Chir 1987;19(1):49–54.

[25] Larsson SE. Compression arthrodesis of the wrist. A consecutive series of 23 cases. Clin Orthop 1974;99:146–53.

[26] Hodgson SP, Stanley JK, Muirhead A. The Wrightington classification of rheumatoid wrist X-rays: a guide to surgical management. J Hand Surg [Br] 1989;14(4):451–5.

[27] Alnot JY, Leroux D. Realignment stabilization synovectomy in the rheumatoid wrist. A study of twenty-five cases. Ann Chir Main 1985;4(4):294–305.

[28] Stanley JK, Hullin MG. Wrist arthrodesis as part of composite surgery of the hand. J Hand Surg [Br] 1986;11(2):243–4.

[29] Stanley JK, Boot DA. Radio-lunate arthrodesis. J Hand Surg [Br] 1989;14(3):283–7.

[30] Alnot JY, Fauroux L. Synovectomy in the realignment-stabilization of the rheumatoid wrist. Apropos of a series of 104 cases with average follow-up of 5 years. Rev Rhum Mal Osteoartic 1992;59(3):196–206.

[31] Borisch N, Lerch K, Grifka J, et al. A comparison of two indices for ulnar translation and carpal height in the rheumatoid wrist. J Hand Surg [Br] 2004;29(2):144–7.

[32] Bouman H-W, Messer E, Sennwald G. Measurement of ulnar translation and carpal height. J Hand Surg [Br] 1994;19:325–9.

[33] Taleisnik J. Combined radiocarpal arthrodesis and midcarpal (lunocapitate) arthroplasty for treatment of rheumatoid arthritis of the wrist. J Hand Surg [Am] 1987;12(1):1–8.

[34] Backdahl M. The caput ulna syndrome in rheumatoid arthritis: a study of the morphology, abnormal anatomy and clinical picture. Acta Rheuma Scand 1963;(Suppl 5):1–8.

[35] Thirupathi RG, Ferlic DC, Clayton ML. Dorsal wrist synovectomy in rheumatoid arthritis—a long-term study. J Hand Surg [Am] 1983;8(6):848–56.

[36] Masada K, Hashimoto H, Yasuda M. Radiographic changes after resection of the distal ulna in patients with rheumatoid arthritis. Scand J Plast Reconstr Surg Hand Surg 2002;36(5):300–4.

[37] Ishikawa H, Hanyu T, Tajima T. Rheumatoid wrists treated with synovectomy of the extensor tendons and the wrist joint combined with a Darrach procedure. J Hand Surg [Am] 1992;17(6):1109–17.

[38] Chantelot C, Fontaine C, Flipo RM, et al. Synovectomy combined with the Sauve-Kapandji procedure for the rheumatoid wrist. J Hand Surg [Br] 1999;24(4):405–9.

[39] Stack HG, Vaughan-Jackson OJ. The zig-zag deformity of the rheumatoid hand. Hand 1971;3:62–7.

[40] Chamay A, Della Santa D, Vilaseca A. Radiolunate arthrodesis. Factor of stability for the rheumatoid wrist. Ann Chir Main 1983;2(1):5–17.

[41] Borisch N, Haussmann P. Radiolunate arthrodesis in the rheumatoid wrist: a retrospective clinical and radiological long-term follow-up. J Hand Surg [Br] 2002;27(1):61–72.

[42] Nalebuff EA, Garrod KJ. Present approach to the severely involved rheumatoid wrist. Orthop Clin North Am 1984;15(2):369–80.

[43] Linscheid RL, Dobyns JH. Radiolunate arthrodesis. J Hand Surg [Am] 1985;10(6 Pt 1):821–9.

[44] Chamay A, Della Santa D. Radiolunate arthrodesis in rheumatoid wrist (21 cases). Ann Chir Main Memb Super 1991;10(3):197–206.

[45] Evans DM, Ansell BM, Hall MA. The wrist in juvenile arthritis. J Hand Surg [Br] 1991;16(3):293–304.

[46] Inoue G, Tamura Y. Radiolunate and radioscapholunate arthrodesis. Arch Orthop Trauma Surg 1992;111(6):333–5.

[47] Ishikawa H, Hanyu T, Saito H, et al. Limited arthrodesis for the rheumatoid wrist. J Hand Surg [Am] 1992;17(6):1103–9.

[48] Della Santa D, Chamay A. Radiological evolution of the rheumatoid wrist after radio-lunate arthrodesis. J Hand Surg [Br] 1995;20(2):146–54.

[49] Halikis MN, Colello-Abraham K, Taleisnik J. Radiolunate fusion. The forgotten partial arthrodesis. Clin Orthop 1997;341:30–5.

[50] Ishikawa H, Murasawa A, Nakazono K. Long-term follow-up study of radiocarpal arthrodesis for the rheumatoid wrist. J Hand Surg [Am] 2005;30:656–66.

[51] Rittmeister M, Kandziora F, Rehart S, et al. Radiolunar Mannerfelt arthrodesis in rheumatoid arthritis. Handchir Mikrochir Plast Chir 1999;31(4):266–73.

[52] Doets HC, Raven EEJ. A procedure for stabilising and preserving mobility in the arthritic wrist. J Bone Joint Surg [Br] 1999;81(6):1013–6.

[53] Schill S, Luhr T, Thabe H. Radiolunate arthrodesis of the rheumatoid wrist—mid- and long-term results. Z Rheumatol 2002;61(5):551–9.

[54] Berger R, Bishop A. A fiber-splitting capsulotomy technique for dorsal exposure of the wrist. Tech Hand Upper Extrem Surg 1997;1:2–10.

ELSEVIER
SAUNDERS

Hand Clin 21 (2005) 553–559

HAND
CLINICS

Proximal Row Carpectomy

Edward Diao, MD*, Allen Andrews, BA, MPhil, McPherson Beall, MD

*Department of Orthopaedic Surgery, University of California San Francisco, 500 Parnassus Avenue,
MU320W, San Francisco, CA 94143-0728, USA*

The origin of proximal row carpectomy was described by David Green to T.T. Stamm of Guy's Hospital in London, who first did the operation in 1939. He credited Lambrinudi with the concept of treating a nonunited fracture of the scaphoid with excision not only of the scaphoid but of the entire proximal row of the carpus. Stamm's first experience was to provide relief for painful degenerative wrist disease without having to resort to arthrodesis or fusion [1].

Stack wrote about carpectomy of just the scaphoid and the lunate in 1948 [2]. In 1964 Crabbe reported on 20 patients treated by Stamm in England between 1943 and 1962. Sixteen of 20 of these results were classified as good, with joint pain relief and retention of a functional range of motion and strength [3]. Warren and Stubbins in 1944 described carpectomy for intractable flexion deformities of the wrists owing to extrinsic causes [4].

Indications

Proximal row carpectomy is a useful procedure for various conditions. It is useful in cases of degenerative joint arthritis regardless of cause, be they idiopathic, osteoarthritis, scapholunate advance collapse, or status post-intercarpal pathology, such as lunate dislocation or transcaphoid perilunate fracture dislocation [5,6]. It has been used for patients who have Kienböck disease and on patients who have rheumatoid arthritis and osteoarthritis [7,8].

Preoperative evaluations are focused on an understanding of the extent of the patient's

disability based on the patient's subjective evaluation of pain and loss of function and on objective evaluations of wrist range of motion and grip strength. Pain is the most common reason to pursue proximal row carpectomy, and pain itself is often a difficult parameter to assess. Using analog pain evaluation instruments and objective findings is at this time the best way to evaluate such patients.

Patients should have had a full complement of conservative treatment measures, including physical therapy modalities, home exercises, intermittent use of mechanical bracing of the wrist, and a trial of anti-inflammatory agents administered orally or by injection.

Imaging studies to evaluate the particulars of the intra-articular pathology of the radiocarpal joint can be helpful but generally are not necessary for preoperative planning if the surgeon is prepared to perform proximal row carpectomy or one of the variations. If there is significant intra-articular pathology on the distal radius, imaging studies can be beneficial to assess the appropriateness of a proximal row carpectomy procedure to ameliorate pain and loss of function. Pathology on the proximal scaphoid, lunate, or triquetrum is less critical, because these bones are sacrificed during the procedure. The state of the proximal pole of the capitate is germane, however. Variations on the standard operation can be performed in the case of distal radius pathology or proximal capitate pathology, including resection with interposition [9] or resection distraction [10].

More recently the senior author has used arthroscopy of the radiocarpal and midcarpal joints to evaluate the joint surfaces before proceeding with the definitive surgery that might involve proximal row carpectomy. Arthroscopic evaluation of serious pathology of the distal

* Corresponding author.

E-mail address: diaoe@orthosurg.ucsf.edu (E. Diao).

0749-0712/05/$ - see front matter © 2005 Elsevier Inc. All rights reserved.
doi:10.1016/j.hcl.2005.08.006

radius or the capitate in loss of cartilage or irregularity can help determine the need for adjunctive procedures in addition to the proximal row resection.

Alternatives to proximal row carpectomy

There are alternatives to treating significant intra-articular wrist pathology besides proximal row carpectomy. Traditionally the most basic procedure is wrist arthrodesis. It has the advantage of removal of joints in the wrist, thereby eliminating the source of mechanical pain, but at the same time sacrifices wrist motion except for pronation and supination. These operations are predictable and durable and can be performed with little regard for the degree of intra-articular pathology or even bone quality. Casts, pins, intermedullary fixation, and plate and screw fixation all work well, and reports of the success of these are well documented in the literature [11–13].

The main bone reconstructive technique that retains motion at the wrist is intercarpal arthrodesis. Several studies have evaluated comparative results of proximal row carpectomy with scaphoid excision and four-corner fusion [14,15]. In these studies, proximal row carpectomy performed as well as, if not somewhat better than, the scaphoid excision and four-corner fusion in patients.

Most recently total wrist arthroplasty is the other alternative to proximal row carpectomy. This topic is discussed by Anderson and Adams elsewhere in this issue.

Surgical technique

Exposure to the dorsum of the distal radius, proximal carpal row, and midcarpal row can be accomplished through a longitudinal or transverse incision. The senior author (ED) prefers the transverse incision for its cosmetic appearance. After incising through the skin, soft tissue dissection is performed carefully, preserving the longitudinally oriented dorsal veins and nerves. Exposure can be facilitated by subperiosteal dissection in the interspace between the third and fourth compartments, centered over Lister tubercle. Alternatively, the fourth compartment itself can be entered. The exposure can be facilitated by placing Penrose drains around the extensor tendons of the first, second, and third compartment to be retracted radialward and around the contents of the fourth compartment to be retracted ulnarward. Capsular exposure is best done through a transverse incision. If interposition of the dorsal capsule is contemplated, then taking the capsule as distally as possible off of the carpal bones is the goal. This can be extended with longitudinal incisions on the radial and the ulnar aspect to form a proximally-based dorsal flap. Allis clamps can be used to retract this dorsal capsule. Excision of the carpal bones then is performed. It is not necessary to keep the bones intact, and removing them in piecemeal fashion is often a more expeditious way to perform this portion of the procedure. Use of osteotomes or curettes can be helpful. The most densely adherent portions of the carpal bones are the attachments to the volar capsule and wrist ligaments. Although some investigators allow maintenance of a shell of carpal bone, the senior author prefers to fully remove the lunate, triquetrum, and proximal pole of scaphoid. The author retains the distal pole of the scaphoid to keep the scaphotrapezial ligaments intact.

After removal of the lunate, triquetrum, and most of the scaphoid, the capitate and the distal radius should be inspected carefully. One can opt for leaving normal articulations in place. Alternatively, a partial resection of the proximal capitate can be performed to improve the matching of the arc of the distal carpal row to the curvature of the radius articular surface, as has been described in Salomon and Eaton's description and in the description by Fitzgerald and colleagues [9,10]. Of course, having normal or preserved articular surfaces obviates the need for this. In the senior author's experience, removal of this proximal capitate bone leads to a better result.

In cases in which the proximal capitate has significant chondromalacia or degenerative joint disease or in which there are arthritic changes in the lunate fossa, the debridement or excision of either or both of these surfaces is indicated.

In general, use of an interposition is beneficial. By retaining a dorsal flap of capsule, this can now be sutured to the volar wrist capsule and wrist ligaments through the resection site using absorbable sutures. In an alternative technique, use of exogenous soft tissue such as autograft or allograft fascia lata or Graft Jacket (Wright Medical; Arlington, TN) can be incorporated into the resection site. The use of transfixing smooth Steinman pins or Kirschner wires is optional.

Resection of the posterior interosseous nerve can be accomplished easily with exposure of the fourth dorsal compartment to aid in pain relief.

The skin can be closed by sutures and the wrist maintained with a dorsal or volar splint for 4 weeks to allow soft tissue healing.

Case 1

A 40-year-old right-hand–dominant man was involved in a motor vehicle accident in Yemen 17 months before presentation in which he sustained a left transradial styloid perilunate dislocation initially treated by open reduction of the dislocation and wire fixation of the radial styloid. The carpus re-dislocated and developed a nonunion of the styloid, leading to persistent pain and stiffness. Examination revealed minimal forearm rotation and wrist motion, and radiographs revealed a chronic dorsal perilunate dislocation with radial styloid nonunion (Fig. 1).

A dorsal surgical approach allowed extensive extensor tenolysis, sectioning of the posterior interosseous nerve, and elevation of the dorsal capsule as a flap for possible interposition. Soft tissue contracture precluded reduction of the dislocation, therefore a proximal row carpectomy was performed with excision of the dorsally displaced scaphoid and triquetrum and the ununited radial styloid fragment. Flexion of the wrist allowed excision of the lunate. The articular surfaces of the proximal capitate and lunate fossa of the radius were in good condition; therefore, interposition of the dorsal capsule was not necessary. Release of the volar soft tissues through the dorsal approach allowed reduction of the capitate to the radius. A tendency toward dorsal instability of the carpus mandated pinning of the capitate to the radius (Fig. 2).

Postoperatively one of the pins was removed at week 3 because of a superficial infection. The remaining pin was removed and active range of motion was started at week 4. Wrist flexion was 45° and extension was 30° with a 180° arc of forearm rotation at the 7-week follow-up visit. Pain was improved compared with preoperative ratings, and no recurrent subluxation or dislocation was noted.

Case 2

A 78-year-old right-hand–dominant man felt a pop in his wrist while using a screwdriver, followed by several years of increasing dorsal wrist pain. Initial range of motion was 45° flexion, 50° extension, 90° pronation, and 90° supination. Radiographs revealed disruption of the scapholunate ligament with scapholunate advanced collapse (Fig. 3). He elected to undergo proximal row carpectomy to prioritize initial range of motion over grip strength.

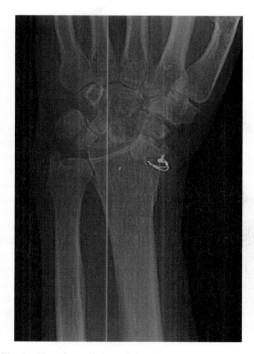

Fig. 1. Chronic perilunate dislocation. Note the triangular appearance of the lunate and the nonunion of the radial styloid.

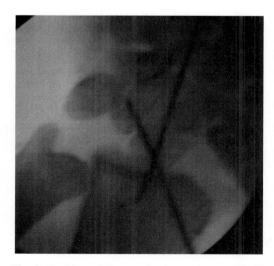

Fig. 2. Excision of the proximal carpal row with K-wires to maintain reduction.

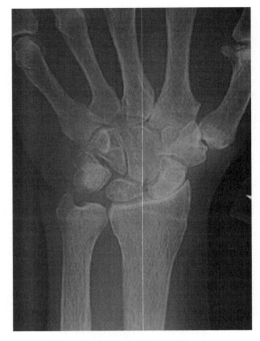

Fig. 3. Early stage III scapholunate advanced collapse.

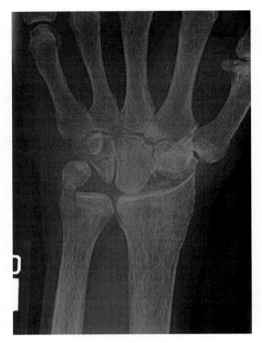

Fig. 4. Settling of the distal row after proximal row carpectomy with styloid impingement on the trapezium.

Through a dorsal approach, the posterior interosseous nerve was sectioned and the wrist capsule was elevated as a proximally-based flap. The proximal row was excised, and degeneration of the proximal capitate articular surface mandated interposition of the dorsal capsular flap (Fig. 4).

Nine months postoperatively he had 30° flexion, 30° extension, and a 180° arc of forearm rotation with persistent pain and dorsal tenderness. Radiographs revealed progressive impingement of the radial styloid against the trapezium. At subsequent wrist arthroscopy the interposition material was found to be intact except over the prominent radial styloid, which was excised through a small radial incision with arthroscopic assistance (Fig. 5). At 4 weeks he had significantly improved pain control and has maintained 30° flexion and 30° extension.

Results

Most literature regarding proximal row carpectomy is comprised of retrospective reviews of clinical series. As previously mentioned, Stack in 1948 reported favorable results in nine wrists of seven patients for perilunate dislocations associated with fracture of the carpal navicular [2]. McLaughlin and Baad had a report on three cases in 1951 [16], and Crabbe reported on 20 cases in his 1964 review with 15 good results, 2 fair results, and 3 failures [3].

The largest series of the modern era starts with a report by Jorgensen. In 1969 Jorgensen and co-authors performed direct retrospective review of 22 proximal row carpectomy cases performed over 20 years. In the cases that contain records of pre- and postoperative wrist motion, there was an increase in motion after surgery. There were no complications, but all patients reported some subjective feeling of weakness [17]. Inglis and James reviewed the Hospital for Special Surgery experience in 1977 [18]. This was a retrospective review of 12 cases. They believed that pain relief and functional range of motion was achieved in all patients without any evidence of progressive degenerative arthritis of the radiocapitate articulation. They did not observe weakness in these patients, and all patients returned to their preoperative occupations. All of their patients had at least 45° of flexion and extension, and 5 of the 12 patients have flexion and extension equal to the contralateral wrist. The investigators also concluded that a mild degree of degenerative arthritis

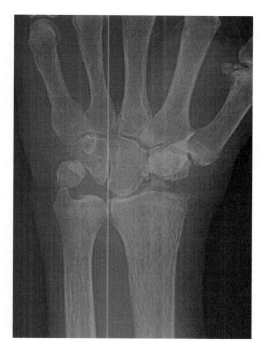

Fig. 5. Status post-arthroscopic–assisted radial styloidectomy. Interposition material was found to be intact except over the styloid.

preoperatively did not preclude good results. In 1983 Neviaser reviewed 24 patients retrospectively. He retained a shell of the cortex in each of the three bones adhering to the palmar capsule, and if the trapezium abutted against the radial styloid, he performed radial styloidectomy. Twenty-three of 24 patients had satisfactory pain relief and range of motion in this 3–10-year follow-up, with one failure in a psychiatric patient. Extension of 45° and flexion of 40° was achieved in the transscaphoid perilunate dislocation group and similar results were obtained for nonunion of scaphoid and scapholunate dissociation groups [6]. Green's study had acceptable results in 13 of 15 patients [1], and Fitzgerald and colleagues' review in 1989 of distraction resection arthroplasty in 14 wrists compared favorably to proximal row carpectomy in 9 patients, with 4 of 23 wrists requiring secondary arthrodesis [10].

Imbriglia and colleagues' review in 1990 of 27 patients, 10 of whom had radial styloidectomies, showed that the postoperative patients all had increased arc of motion except for radial deviation, with 26 of 27 patients having excellent pain relief requiring no medicines or splints postoperatively, and 24 of 27 patients returning to previous

activities within an average of 4.5 months after surgery. For vigorous manual labor, 16 of 19 of these were able to return to their previous occupation. Range of motion improved over preoperative conditions in all patients, and grip strength was improved compared with the contralateral side. Two re-operations were required for secondary radial styloidectomy and one patient with persistent pain had wrist fusion [19].

Ferlic and colleagues in 1991 reviewed 18 patients, 9 who had rheumatoid arthritis and 9 who had nonrheumatoid arthritis who received proximal row carpectomy procedures. There were contrasts between the two groups, with six of eight patients who had nonrheumatoid arthritis with satisfactory results and two failures treated with wrist fusion. The patients who had rheumatoid arthritis had only two of eight wrists that were satisfactory [20]. In a review of patients treated with proximal row carpectomy for Kienböck disease, Lin and Stern compared proximal row carpectomy and wrist arthrodesis, and both had generally excellent results [21]. Culp and colleagues' multicenter study in 1993 saw 83% return to work [8]. There was some decrease in range of motion, but grip strength increased. Overall 82% of patients had satisfactory results. Most patients in this series had post-traumatic arthritis. An interesting study by Krakauer and colleagues in 1994 compared different reconstructive procedures for scapholunate advanced collapse in 55 cases [22]. Of these, 12 cases of proximal row carpectomy were evaluated. They concluded that proximal row carpectomy was the best procedure in preservation of mobility, flexion extension arcs, and reasonable satisfaction in pain relief. Begley and colleagues' 1994 review looked at 16 patients with proximal row carpectomy to treat Kienböck disease with one excellent, nine good, and four fair clinical results using the Glickel/Millender scale [7]. Tomaino and colleagues' review in 1994 of 23 wrists were performed with retention of the distal scaphoid in two patients and no internal fixation. Radial styloidectomies were performed in three patients, and one case of interposition technique was used. Twenty of 23 patients had good satisfaction with functional performance and pain relief. There were two failures and one additional patient who had progressive radiocarpal degeneration postsurgery. Sixty-one percent of contralateral side wrist motion and 79% grip strength of contralateral side was noted [23].

Salomon's review of Eaton's series of 12 proximal row carpectomy patients with partial capitate resection had seven patients with no postoperative pain and four patients with occasional pain with strenuous activity. Arc of motion increased from 80° preoperatively to 94° postoperatively with improvement of grip strength from 19 kg to 26 kg. All of the patients returned to their preoperative occupation [9].

Rettig and Raskin's 1999 review of 12 patients who had chronic perilunate dislocations revealed excellent results with 9 patients with no pain and 3 with mild pain after heavy use. Restoration of range of motion and grip strength was achieved, with an average range of motion of 45° flexion, 35° extension, and grip strength 80% of the contralateral side. Eight patients returned to previous employment, and three were unable to return to their previous occupation [5].

Culp's review of 17 patients, 5 with scaphoid nonunion advanced collapse and 12 with scapholunate advanced collapse, excluded patients with severe capitate to lunate fossa arthritic changes. Both groups had similar outcomes in range of motion, grip strength, and overall efficacy, with most patients in the good to excellent category [8]. In Didonna and colleagues' review in 2004, 22 patients who had proximal row carpectomy were reviewed with a minimum 10-year follow-up [24]. Ten of 22 patients had radial styloidectomy and some had Kirschner wire or temporary fixation that was abandoned in the later patients because of complications, including pin-track infections. Four of 22 patients had failures at an average of 7 years or in patients who were younger than 35 years old at the time of proximal row carpectomy. The average flexion extension arc was 72°, and average grip strength was 91% of the contralateral side. Fourteen of 18 were very satisfied and 4 were satisfied. These investigators concluded that caution should be exercised in using proximal row carpectomy in patients younger than 35 years old. Additionally, they believed that degeneration of the radiocapitate joint, which was seen in 14 wrists, did not preclude an excellent clinical result following conventional proximal row carpectomy. Jebson and colleagues' review in 2003 of 20 patients showed 2 with failures requiring radiocapitate arthrodesis [25]. The other 18 were followed for an average of 13.1 years. Seventeen of 18 were satisfied with the outcome. The one who was not satisfied because of persistent pain did not seek further surgery. Sixteen of 20 patients returned to their previous occupation, average wrist range of motion was 63%, and average grip strength was 83% of the contralateral side.

Follow-up radiographs showed some proximal capitate changes in 6 of 20 patients.

In summary, all reviews revealed that patients receiving proximal row carpectomy had excellent functional results. The exceptions were patients who had rheumatoid disease and those younger than 35 years of age. Additionally, the two studies that reviewed proximal row carpectomy versus four-corner fusion found the proximal row carpectomy to be as good as or slightly better than the intercarpal arthrodesis patients [14,15].

Summary

Proximal row carpectomy is extremely useful as a wrist reconstructive technique for cases of degenerative joint arthritis of the radiocarpal joint caused by scapholunate advanced collapse, scaphoid nonunion advanced collapse, trans-scaphoid perilunate fracture dislocations, lunate dislocations, and Kienböck disease. It should be selected with caution for patients who have rheumatoid arthritis or for patients younger than 35 years old. The procedure can be performed with or without temporary internal fixation with Kirschner wires, and adjunctive techniques of dorsal capsule interposition, proximal capitate excision, and radial styloidectomy can be used. The longevity of the operation is good, but the patient should be informed preoperatively that secondary procedures may be required. Based on historical series, these procedures have included addition of radial styloidectomy when this has not been performed at the index procedure, revision of the surgery with capitate debridement or additional interposition material, or conversion to total wrist arthrodesis. Conversion of proximal row carpectomy to total wrist arthroplasty with implants can be contemplated in selected patients, particularly as newer implants are designed.

The technique the senior author has used on occasion has been to use arthroscopy and arthroscopic procedures to perform revision surgery on those patients who have chronic pain who might need further debridement of the radius, in the radial styloid, the proximal capitate, or evaluation of the integrity of the interposition.

Supplemental procedures

As use of wrist arthroscopy is widespread, the wrist arthroscope can be used as an adjunct to proximal row carpectomy. It can be performed as a preoperative staging procedure to assess the condition of the proximal capitate and the distal radius, to identify the supplemental techniques that may be appropriate in performing a subsequent proximal row carpectomy, or if the surgeon chooses not to use these adjunctive procedures, to aid the selection of an alternative wrist salvage procedure.

Alternatively, in situations in which a proximal row carpectomy has been performed and there may be some residual pain, the arthroscopy can be used to evaluate the status of the proximal capitate, the distal radial articular surface, and the condition of any interposition material that may have been introduced during the index procedure, as illustrated in case 2.

References

[1] Green DP. Proximal row carpectomy. Hand Clin 1987;3(1):163–8.

[2] Stack JK. End results of excision for the carpal bones. Arch Surg 1948;57:245–52.

[3] Crabbe WA. Excision of the proximal row of the carpus. J Bone Joint Surg [Br] 1964;46:708–11.

[4] Warren WJ, Stubbins SG. Carpectomy for intractable flexion deformities of the wrist. J Bone Joint Surg [Am] 1944;26:131–8.

[5] Rettig ME, Raskin KB. Long-term assessment of proximal row carpectomy for chronic perilunate dislocations. J Hand Surg [Am] 1999;24(6):1231–6.

[6] Neviaser RJ. Proximal row carpectomy for posttraumatic disorders of the carpus. J Hand Surg [Am] 1983;8(3):301–5.

[7] Begley BW, Engber WD. Proximal row carpectomy in advanced Kienböck's disease. J Hand Surg [Am] 1994;19(6):1016–8.

[8] Culp RW, McGuigan FX, Turner MA, et al. Proximal row carpectomy: a multicenter study. J Hand Surg [Am] 1993;18(1):19–25.

[9] Salomon GD, Eaton RG. Proximal row carpectomy with partial capitate resection. J Hand Surg [Am] 1996;21(1):2–8.

[10] Fitzgerald JP, Peim CA, Smith RJ, et al. Distraction resection arthroplasty of the wrist. J Hand Surg [Am] 1989;14(5):774–81.

[11] Haddad RJ Jr, Riordan DC. Arthrodesis of the wrist. A surgical technique. J Bone Joint Surg [Am] 1967;49(5):950–4.

[12] Hastings H 2nd, Weiss AP, Quenzer D, et al. Arthrodesis of the wrist for post-traumatic disorders. J Bone Joint Surg [Am] 1996;78(6):897–902.

[13] Wood MB. Wrist arthrodesis using dorsal radial bone graft. J Hand Surg [Am] 1987;12(2):208–12.

[14] Cohen MS, Kozin SH. Degenerative arthritis of the wrist: proximal row carpectomy versus scaphoid excision and four-corner arthrodesis. J Hand Surg [Am] 2001;26(1):94–104.

[15] Wyrick JD, Stern PJ, Kiefhaber TR. Motion-preserving procedures in the treatment of scapholunate advanced collapse wrist: proximal row carpectomy versus four-corner arthrodesis. J Hand Surg [Am] 1995;20(6):965–70.

[16] McLaughlin HL, Baab OD. Carpectomy. Surg Clin North Am 1951;31:451–61.

[17] Jorgensen EC. Proximal-row carpectomy. An end-result study of twenty-two cases. J Bone Joint Surg [Am] 1969;51(6):1104–11.

[18] Inglis AE, Jones EC. Proximal-row carpectomy for diseases of the proximal row. J Bone Joint Surg [Am] 1977;59(4):460–3.

[19] Imbriglia JE, Broudy AS, Hagberg WC, et al. Proximal row carpectomy: clinical evaluation. J Hand Surg [Am] 1990;15(3):426–30.

[20] Ferlic DC, Clayton ML, Mills MF. Proximal row carpectomy: review of rheumatoid and nonrheumatoid wrists. J Hand Surg [Am] 1991;16(3):420–4.

[21] Lin HH, Stern PJ. "Salvage" procedures in the treatment of Kienböck's disease. Proximal row carpectomy and total wrist arthrodesis. Hand Clin 1993;9(3):521–6.

[22] Krakauer JD, Bishop AT, Conney WP. Surgical treatment of scapholunate advanced collapse. J Hand Surg [Am] 1994;19(5):751–9.

[23] Tomaino MM, Delsignore J, Burton RI. Long-term results following proximal row carpectomy. J Hand Surg [Am] 1994;19(4):694–703.

[24] DiDonna ML, Kiefhaber TR, Stern PJ. Proximal row carpectomy: study with a minimum of ten years of follow-up. J Bone Joint Surg [Am] 2004;86A(11):2359–65.

[25] Jebson PJ, Hayes EP, Engber WD. Proximal row carpectomy: a minimum 10-year follow-up study. J Hand Surg [Am] 2003;28(4):561–9.

Radioscapholunate Arthrodesis

Peter M. Murray, MD[a,b,*]

[a]Division of Hand and Microvascular Surgery, Department of Orthopaedic Surgery,
Mayo Graduate School of Medicine, 200 1st SW, Rochester, MN 52242, USA
[b]Hand and Microvascular Surgery, Department of Orthopaedic Surgery,
Mayo Clinic, 4500 San Pablo Road, Jacksonville, FL 32224, USA

Fractures of the distal radius extending into the radiocarpal joint that head with greater than a 2-mm step-off have been shown to be at greater risk for posttraumatic degenerative arthritis, leading to pain and functional limitations [1]. Similarly, radiocarpal destruction from systemic inflammatory arthritis can cause pain and limit upper extremity function. High fusion rates and good pain relief can be expected with complete wrist arthrodesis, but many patients may find the loss of motion limiting. Most activities of daily living can be accomplished with wrist motion in the range of 10° flexion, 35° extension, 10° radial deviation, and 15° ulnar deviation [2], indicating that preservation of partial motion is a worthwhile goal. Although wrist replacement arthroplasty can restore a pain-free functional arc of motion, it is not a durable option for patients who have high physical demands.

In 1961 Gordon and King reported the first experience with radioscapholunate arthrodesis (RSL) [3]. Although RSL arthrodesis is an intuitively appealing option for arthritis limited to the radiocarpal joint, little has been published on the topic. A successful radioscapholunate arthrodesis is predicated on having a nearly normal midcarpal joint. Despite previous reports of high complication rates for limited arthrodesis procedures in the wrist [4], degenerative or inflammatory arthritis found isolated to the radiocarpal articulation presents the surgical option for an RSL arthrodesis to preserve some wrist motion. The purpose of this article is to review the kinematics, technique, and results of RSL arthrodesis.

Kinematics

Traditionally, the flexion/extension arc of wrist range of motion was considered equally divided between the radiocarpal and midcarpal joints. Nalebuff and colleagues commented that only 25%–50% of preoperative range of motion can be expected following RSL arthrodesis [5]. Ruby and colleagues, using a cadaver model, concluded that the wrist functions as two separate joints, with flexion and extension derived equally from the two articulations [6]. Gellmann and colleagues found in a cadaver model that 63% of wrist flexion and 53% of wrist extension occurred at the proximal carpal row [7]. In contrast, Kobayashi and colleagues found, using 22 cadaver specimens under physiologic loading, radiocarpal motion accounted for 50% of wrist extension but only 36% of wrist flexion [8]. In seven normal cadaver wrists and three cadaver wrists with scapholunate disruption, Wolfe and colleagues, using CT analysis, determined that in the normal state the relative contributions of the radiocarpal and midcarpal joints to wrist flexion and extension were equal [9]. With disruption of the scapholunate interosseous ligament, however, the midcarpal joint provided 57% of wrist flexion/extension range of motion [9]. This implies synergy of motion from the radiocarpal and midcarpal joints as it relates to wrist flexion and extension. More recently, Wolfe and colleagues have shown in an in vivo model that the scaphoid contribution to global wrist flexion and extension is greater than once

* Division of Hand and Microvascular Surgery, Department of Orthopaedic Surgery, Mayo Clinic, 4500 San Pablo Road, Jacksonville, FL 32224, USA.

E-mail address: murray.peter@mayo.edu

believed (Fig. 1) [10]. In wrist flexion, the scaphoid measured 73% of capitate flexion and 46% of the lunate [10]. In extension, the scaphoid measured 99% of capitate extension. This relative scapholunate motion and out-of-plane scaphoid rotation [10] during wrist flexion and extension may account for the less than expected wrist motion obtained following arthrodesis of the proximal carpal row to the distal radius.

Indications

Radiocarpal joint degeneration can result from posttraumatic arthritis, inflammatory arthritis, or osteoarthritis. Knirk and Jupiter [1] have shown that in young patients who have distal radius fractures, 91% of fractures healing with radiocarpal joint incongruity go on to degenerative arthritis. In these patients degenerative arthritis of the lunate fossa articulation may be all that is involved, with the remainder of the radiocarpal joint being normal (Fig. 2). This is a key distinguishing feature from the more common form of degenerative wrist arthritis, scapholunate advanced collapse (SLAC) (Fig. 3). In stage III SLAC wrist the entire radioscaphoid articulation and the capitolunate articulation have degenerative changes, whereas the radiolunate joint is preserved. When

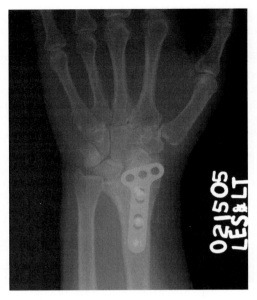

Fig. 2. A 47-year-old woman with posttraumatic degenerative arthritis of the radiocarpal joint following an intra-articular left distal radius fracture.

patients who have radiocarpal arthritis become symptomatic, nonoperative measures are advised first. Modalities such as wrist splinting, radiocarpal injection, nonsteroidal anti-inflammatory agents, ultrasound, paraffin wax treatments, and

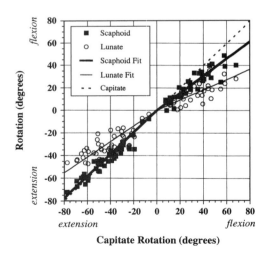

Fig. 1. Graphic demonstration of scaphoid and lunate contribution to wrist flexion and extension range of motion. Wrist flexion and extension defined as capitate rotation. (*From* Wolfe et al. In vivo scaphoid, lunate and capitate kinematics in flexion and in extension. J Hand Surg [Am] 2000;25(5):864; with permission.)

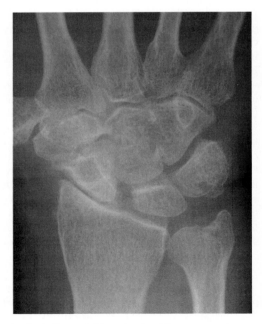

Fig. 3. A 53-year-old mechanic with symptomatic stage II scapholunate advanced collapse (SLAC) wrist.

galvanic stimulation may prove useful in certain patients. Long-term relief from these modalities is, however, unlikely.

Although isolated radiocarpal degenerative arthritis exists in patients who have stage I or stage II SLAC wrists (Fig. 3) and fusion of the radiocarpal joint is an alternative [11], other surgical options are used more commonly. Procedures such as proximal row carpectomy, scaphoidectomy, radial styloidectomy, and four-corner fusion make use of the preserved radiolunate articulation [12–14].

In certain instances, patients who have rheumatoid arthritis or other inflammatory arthritic conditions may benefit from limited radiocarpal arthrodesis [15]. In these patients the inflammatory synovitis may affect preferentially the radiocarpal joint, leaving the midcarpal joint spared. In the younger, more active rheumatoid patient, the option of an RSL arthrodesis can be considered to preserve midcarpal motion. This is an appealing option for the patient who has rheumatoid arthritis, because it maintains the potential for the tenodesis effect to enhance grip and pinch strength, particularly if tendon transfers for the digits become necessary.

Patients who have stage IV Kienbock have radiocarpal arthritis. These patients have been treated successfully by RSL arthrodesis [16]; however, complete wrist arthrodesis or proximal row carpectomy are used more commonly [17].

second dorsal extensor tendon compartment, follows the distal rim of the radius to Lister tubercle, and then follows the dorsal radiocarpal ligament in line with its fibers. The distal edge of the flap follows the dorsal intercarpal ligament, also in line with its fibers. The dorsal rim of the distal radius can be removed to enhance visualization. The wrist is hyperflexed to expose the opposing articular surfaces of the scaphoid, lunate, and distal radius. The articular cartilage is removed and some areas of subchondral bone are breached to expose cancellous bone for more rapid and complete fusion. The surfaces are contoured to maximize bone opposition between the scaphoid, lunate, and radius. Various implants and fixation techniques can be used, depending on the amount and quality of bone and surgeon preference. Common techniques are percutaneous K-wires (Fig. 4), a low-profile T-plate (Fig. 5), or staples (Fig. 6). Voids between the bones often remain despite contouring. In these circumstances, bone graft from the distal radius, olecranon, or the iliac crest is harvested to supplement the fusion. Alternatively, bone substitute material may be used if the bone quality of the scaphoid, lunate, and radius are not poor, as bone substitutes may not perform as well as autograft. Distal scaphoid excision is considered to enhance postoperative wrist flexion–extension. In a cadaver model, McCombe

Technique

A general or regional anesthetic is used. An indwelling anesthetic catheter can provide prolonged pain relief. The wrist joint is approached through a dorsal midline skin incision. The third and fourth dorsal compartments are identified and the fourth dorsal compartment is elevated ulnarly from the radius in a subperiosteal fashion. The posterior interosseous nerve (PIN) is identified easily in the floor of the fourth dorsal compartment. The anterior interosseous nerve (AIN) can be found just anterior to the interosseous membrane of the forearm. PIN and AIN neurectomies typically are performed according to the technique of Weinstein and Berger to enhance the pain relief of the procedure [18]. The author prefers to expose the joint using a dorsal–radial-based capsular flap, which is intended to preserve the dorsal intercarpal and dorsal radiocarpal ligaments [19]. Its proximal edge begins under the

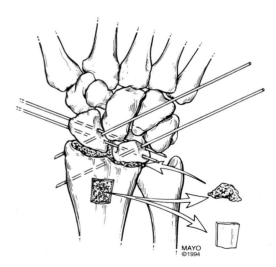

Fig. 4. Technique of radio-scapho-lunate arthrodesis using percutaneous K-wire fixation. (Courtesy of the Mayo Clinic.)

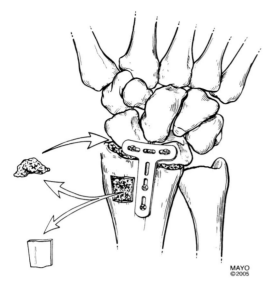

Fig. 5. Technique of radio-scapho-lunate arthrodesis using a low-profile T-plate. (Courtesy of the Mayo Clinic.)

and colleagues [20] showed that distal scaphoid excision following RSL arthrodesis results in increased total passive midcarpal motion from 60° to 122°, which represented 86% of the original wrist motion.

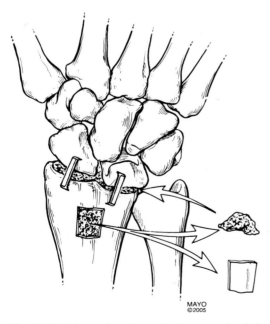

Fig. 6. Technique of radio-scapho-lunate arthrodesis using staples. (Courtesy of the Mayo Clinic.)

Postoperative immobilization includes a cast for approximately 8 weeks followed by conversion to a removable, custom-made splint. Length of cast immobilization depends partially on radiographic evidence of fusion, although it is often difficult to assess the fusion site. If K-wires were used for fixation of the fusion, they are removed at this time. The patient can initiate active and active-assisted range of motion of the wrist once radiographic union had been achieved. Solid radiographic fusion may not be observed for 3 months postoperatively.

Clinical outcome information of RSL arthrodesis is limited, with the largest series having follow-up on 18 patients [21]. Of the RSL series published, the longest single patient follow-up is 11.3 years [22]. Although generally good results have been reported, complications are notable, including pain, early degeneration of the midcarpal joint, fracture of the scaphoid, and nonunion of the arthrodesis [16,22,23].

In the first reported series of RSL fusion, Gordon and King reported on seven patients [3]; four patients had a pre-existing scaphoid nonunion. All patients were reported as pain free at follow-up and all had satisfactory function. Similarly, in 1967 Schwartz reported on five RSL arthrodesis for isolated radiocarpal arthritis, all with a reported good result.

Bach and colleagues [21] have reported the largest experience with RSL fusion. In 36 patients, seven of the cases failed and were converted to complete wrist arthrodesis. Midcarpal arthritis or a history of scaphoid nonunion predisposed to failure. At follow-up, 18 patients had a mean of 48° total active motion. Grip strength was 70% of the contralateral side. Approximately 50% of the patients returned to their original occupation. The investigators concluded that functional result following RSL fusion is generally good as long as the patient is free of midcarpal arthritis.

Beryermann and colleagues [24] reviewed 22 patients who had RSL fusion at an average follow-up of 18.7 months. Their technique included K-wire fixation and cast immobilization for 8 weeks. Average postoperative range of motion was 23° flexion, 24° extension, 9° radial deviation, and 16° ulnar deviation. On average, total range of flexion and extension decreased 21° from preoperative. Average grip strength was 51% of the contralateral side; however, it was improved from preoperative. Pain was decreased in all but one patient. One nonunion occurred. The investigators concluded that RSL fusion was a good alternative for radiocarpal arthritis. Nagy and Buchler reported an average 8-year follow-up on 15 patients who had an RSL arthrodesis for the treatment of posttraumatic arthritis of the radiocarpal joint [22]. Union could not be achieved in four patients and they developed painful carpal instability. Of the 11 patients with a solid RSL arthrodesis, 3 developed early painful midcarpal arthritis. Sturzenegger and Buchler [23] reported a 35.7% incidence of secondary degenerative changes in the midcarpal joint following RSL arthrodesis for posttraumatic arthritis of the radiocarpal joint. In a later report on the same cohort at an average 8-year follow-up, they reviewed the results of 15 patients who had RSL arthrodesis [22]. Union could not be achieved in four patients, and these patients went on to develop painful carpal instability. Of the 11 patients with a solid RSL arthrodesis, 3 developed early painful midcarpal arthritis.

Two patients in the longer-term follow-up surprisingly developed late scaphoid fractures, presumably caused by shearing forces that develop from a rigidly fixed scaphoid on the distal radius [22]. Grip strength averaged 63% of the contralateral side. Average range of motion was 18° flexion, 32° flexion, 3° radial deviation, and 25° ulnar deviation. The investigators judged that seven patients achieved a good, durable result over an average 8-year follow-up period, most in the face of heavy labor occupations. The investigators concluded that patients who had less than two operations before RSL fusion and those who had a preoperative stiff wrist are better candidates for RSL arthrodesis.

Inoue and Tamura [16] reported on 11 patients who had degenerative wrist arthritis treated with limited wrist fusions. Four patients received an RSL fusion. All four patients achieved union and all were relieved of pain. Range of motion improved in all patients and grip strength improved at least threefold.

Ishikawa and colleagues reported good results for nine RSL arthrodeses in patients who had rheumatoid arthritis [15]. These results were reported as part of a group of 25 patients, 16 who had radiolunate arthrodesis. Although the investigators did not distinguish data based on the type of fusion, pain relief and improved grip strength occurred in all patients. Wrist flexion and extension decreased from preoperative. At an average 3-year follow-up, midcarpal deterioration was noted in one half of the wrists.

Summary

Although RSL fusion is a viable option for isolated radiocarpal arthritis, the enthusiasm for this procedure should be tempered with the reality that kinematics of the wrist is not entirely suited for independent midcarpal flexion and extension [10]. Limited wrist flexion and extension is expected following a successful RSL arthrodesis. The effects of imposed abnormal kinematics are further shown by the high incidence of RSL nonunions, occurrence of scaphoid fractures, and postoperative deterioration of the midcarpal joint [15,22]. In a young patient with posttraumatic arthritis or rheumatoid arthritis limited to the radiocarpal joint, however, RSL arthrodesis remains a viable alternative to complete wrist arthrodesis if the midcarpal joint is normal. Internal fixation with plates and screws and distal scaphoid excision are technical alternatives to consider when an RSL arthrodesis is performed.

References

[1] Knirk JL, Jupiter JB. Intra-articular fractures of the distal end of the radius in young adults. J Bone Joint Surg [Am] 1986;68(5):647–59.

[2] Palmer AK, Werner FW, Murphy D, et al. Functional wrist motion: a biomechanical study. J Hand Surg [Am] 1985;10(1):39–46.

[3] Gordon LH, King D. Partial wrist arthrodesis for old un-united fractures of the carpal navicular. Am J Surg 1961;102:460–4.

[4] McAuliffe JA, Dell PC, Jaffe R. Complications of intercarpal arthrodesis. J Hand Surg [Am] 1993; 18(6):1121–8.

[5] Nalebuff EA, Feldon PG, Millender LH. Rheumatoid arthritis in the hand and wrist. In: Green DP, editor. Operative hand surgery. 2nd edition. New York: Churchill Livingstone; 1988. p. 1655–766.

[6] Ruby LK, Cooney WP III, An KN, et al. Relative motion of selected carpal bones: a kinematic analysis of the normal wrist. J Hand Surg [Am] 1988;13(1): 1–10.

[7] Gellman H, Kauffman D, Lenihan M, et al. An in vitro analysis of wrist motion: the effect of limited intercarpal arthrodesis and the contributions of the radiocarpal and midcarpal joints. J Hand Surg [Am] 1988;13(3):378–83.

[8] Kobayashi M, Berger RA, Nagy L, et al. Normal kinematics of carpal bones: a three-dimensional analysis of carpal bone motion relative to the radius. J Biomech 1997;30(8):787–93.

[9] Wolfe SW, Crisco JJ, Katz LD. A non-invasive method for studying in vivo carpal kinematics. J Hand Surg [Br] 1997;22(2):147–52.

[10] Wolfe SW, Neu C, Crisco JJ. In vivo scaphoid, lunate, and capitate kinematics in flexion and in extension. J Hand Surg [Am] 2000;25(5):860–9.

[11] Krakauer JD, Bishop AT, Cooney WP. Surgical treatment of scapholunate advanced collapse. J Hand Surg [Am] 1994;19(5):751–9.

[12] Jebson PJ, Hayes EP, Engber WD. Proximal row carpectomy: a minimum 10-year follow-up study. J Hand Surg [Am] 2003;28(4):561–9.

[13] Hogan CJ, McKay PL, Degnan GG. Changes in radiocarpal loading characteristics after proximal row carpectomy. J Hand Surg [Am] 2004;29(6):1109–13.

[14] Tomaino MM, Delsignore J, Burton RI. Long-term results following proximal row carpectomy. J Hand Surg [Am] 1994;19(4):694–704.

[15] Ishikawa H, Hanyu T, Saito H, et al. Limited arthrodesis for the rheumatoid wrist. J Hand Surg [Am] 1992;17(6):1103–9.

[16] Inoue G, Tamura Y. Radiolunate and radioscapholunate arthrodesis. Arch Orthop Trauma Surg 1992; 111(6):333–5.

[17] Berger RA, Weiss A-PC. Hand surgery. In: Hand surgery. Philadelphia: Lippincott Williams & Wilkins; 2004.

[18] Weinstein LP, Berger RA. Analgesic benefit, functional outcome, and patient satisfaction after partial wrist denervation. J Hand Surg [Am] 2002;27(5): 833–9.

[19] Berger RA, Bishop AT, Bettinger PC. New dorsal capsulotomy for the surgical exposure of the wrist. Ann Plast Surg 1995;35(1):54–9.

[20] McCombe D, Ireland DC, McNab I. Distal scaphoid excision after radioscaphoid arthrodesis. J Hand Surg [Am] 2001;26(5):877–82.

[21] Bach AW, Almquist EE, Newman DM. Proximal row fusion as a solution for radiocarpal arthritis. J Hand Surg [Am] 1991;16(3):424–31.

[22] Nagy L, Buchler U. Long-term results of radioscapholunate fusion following fractures of the distal radius. J Hand Surg [Br] 1997;22(6):705–10.

[23] Sturzenegger M, Buchler U. Radio-scapho-lunate partial wrist arthrodesis following comminuted fractures of the distal radius. Ann Chir Main Memb Super 1991;10(3):207–16.

[24] Beyermann K, Prommesberger K-J, Lanz U. Radioscapholunate fusion following comminuted fractures of the distal radius. Eur J Trauma 2000; 26(4):127–43.

Ulnar Impaction Syndrome

Matthew M. Tomaino, MD, MBA*, John Elfar, MD

Division of Hand, Shoulder and Elbow Surgery, Department of Orthopaedics, University of Rochester Medical Center, 601 Elmwood Avenue, Rochester, NY 14642, USA

Ulnar impaction syndrome is a common degenerative cause of ulnar wrist pain, which develops because of the effects of force transmission across the ulnocarpal joint. Although the pathologic changes and clinical syndrome most typically occur in wrists with ulnar positive variance, ulnar impaction occurs in wrists with ulnar neutral and negative variance also. The diagnosis relies largely on clinical examination and radiographic analysis, and effective treatment, whereas traditionally relying on ulnar shortening osteotomy and open wafer resection increasingly is afforded by arthroscopic decompression.

The ulnar impaction syndrome refers to a painful overload of the ulnocarpal joint [1,2] and has been classified based on pathoanatomy [3] (Table 1). Palmer and Werner have shown that positive ulnar variance results in an increase in ulnocarpal load [4], and this has been implicated in the etiology of degenerative triangular fibrocartilage complex (TFCC) tears [4,5]. Because dynamic increases in ulnar variance may occur with forearm pronation and grip, however [6–8], and an inverse relationship may exist between TFCC thickness and ulnar variance [9], this syndrome also develops in the wrists with neutral or negative ulnar variance [10]. Further, it is known that TFCC wear and undersurface fibrillation occur clinically before perforation [11], and that innervation of the TFCC may, in part, explain pain early in the pathologic spectrum of this condition [12]. Indeed, Palmer's classification of ulnar

impaction accounts for the existence of TFCC wear without central disc perforation [3].

This article addresses the biomechanical bases for treatment options, highlights the authors' pearls regarding examination and diagnosis, and details the surgical options, in particular, the authors' preference—arthroscopic wafer resection of the distal ulna.

Biomechanics

Palmer and Werner have shown that in the ulnar neutral wrist, 80% of the load is transferred across the radiocarpal joint as compared with 20% across the ulnocarpal joint [4]. When variance increases from neutral to 2.5 cm positive, however, ulnocarpal load increases by approximately 20%. Decreasing variance by 2.5 cm lowers force transmission from 20% in the neutral variant to 5%.

These data provide a basis for treating ulnar impaction syndrome with a shortening osteotomy of the ulna [1,2]. Feldon advocated a wafer resection as an alternative in 1992 [13], and in that same year Wnorowski and colleagues showed that an arthroscopic wafer procedure successfully diminished load across the ulnocarpal joint [14]. Most recently, Markolf and colleagues have shown that wafer resection decreases distal ulna forces under all conditions of ulnar variance, although less effectively when variance exceeds 4 mm positive [15].

Although Palmer and Werner have shown that increasing ulnar length results in an increase in force transmission across the distal ulna, and it is known that forearm pronation and forceful grip increase ulnar variance [5,16,17], few studies have investigated loads across the distal ulna when the

_____

* Corresponding author.

E-mail address: matthew_tomaino@urmc.rochester.edu (M.M. Tomaino).

Table 1
Classification of traumatic and degenerative conditions
of the TFCC

Class I – Traumatic
  A. Central perforation
  B. Medial avulsion (ulnar attachment)
    With distal ulnar fracture
    Without distal ulnar fracture
  C. Distal avulsion (carpal attachment)
  D. Lateral avulsion (radial attachment)
    With sigmoid notch fracture
    Without sigmoid notch fracture
Class II – Degenerative (ulnocarpal impaction
  syndrome)
  A. TFCC wear
  B. TFCC wear
    + lunate and/or ulnar chondromalacia
  C. TFCC perforation
    + lunate and/or ulnar chondromalacia
  D. TFCC perforation
    + lunate and/or ulnar chondromalacia
    + L-T ligament perforation
  E. TFCC perforation
    + lunate and/or ulnar chondromalacia
    + L-T ligament perforation
    + ulnocarpal arthritis

forearm is pronated [18,19]. In nine cadaver specimens in different wrist and forearm positions, Glisson and colleagues showed that loads across the distal ulna increased in pronation, wrist flexion, and ulnar deviation [18]. Pfaeffle and colleagues evaluated the effect of axial load and forearm pronation on ulnar variance and distal ulna load in seven cadaver forearms [19]. They found that ulnar variance increased an average of 2 mm in four ulnar positive and three ulnar neutral specimens. Distal ulna load increased in the ulnar neutral wrists and decreased in the ulnar positive wrists in which greater dorsal subluxation of the distal radioulnar joint occurred.

Accurate measurement of variance is therefore important when addressing ulnar wrist pain, because the radioulnar length relationship has profound impact on load transfer across the wrist [20].

Diagnosis

The current diagnostic work-up for ulnar impaction syndrome revolves around the physical examination and plain radiographs. Patients typically complain of ulnar wrist pain; thus, an evaluation of the ulnocarpal and distal radioulnar joint is required. One must evaluate the TFCC,

lunotriquetral (LT) ligament, extensor carpi ulnaris (ECU), flexor carpi ulnaris (FCU) tendons, the pisotriquetral joint, and one must assess for the presence of a midcarpal clunk.

Nakamura's ulnar stress test is performed routinely by deviating ulnarly the pronated wrist while axially loading, flexing, and extending [21] (Fig. 1). The fovea test is performed by asking the patient to flex the wrist. This allows palpation of the FCU, which facilitates locating the fovea of the TFCC—between the FCU and ulnar styloid process. Positive ulnar stress and fovea tests in combination are roughly 98% sensitive in correlation with an objective problem with the TFCC or LT ligament. Exclusion of other sources of discomfort, such as pisotriquetral arthritis, distal radioulnar joint (DRUJ) instability or arthritis, or ECU tendonitis or hypermobility, heightens the suspicion for pathology. History becomes important in hypothesizing the presence of a class I (traumatic) or class II (degenerative) problem with the TFCC. A radiograph series then is obtained to evaluate ulnar variance and to assess for the presence of cystic changes in the ulnar corner of the lunate.

Imaging

Various methods for measuring ulnar variance have been described, but each uses neutral

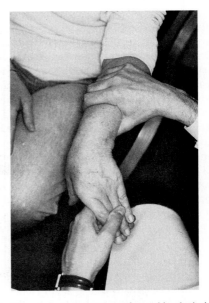

Fig. 1. The ulnar stress test is performed by deviating ulnarly the pronated wrist to provoke ulnar wrist pain caused by TFCC pathology.

rotation posteroanterior (PA) radiographs of the wrist [5,20,22], because pronation slightly increases the length of the ulna. The authors routinely check a zero-rotation PA and lateral view, together with a pronated-grip radiograph taken with the patient making a fist of maximum intensity while the forearm is in pronation [16]. This radiograph may reveal positive ulnar variance not present on a neutral rotation radiograph because of dynamic changes in length when radial shortening occurs during forceful grip [16,17] (Fig. 2).

Why a pronated-grip radiograph? Minami and colleagues were the first to report using such a view, and they showed that positive ulnar variance was associated with poorer outcome following TFCC debridement alone [23]. Their suggestion that persistent pain was related to positive ulnar variance is consistent with the message of two other reports that have shown the efficacy of ulnar shortening osteotomy in two situations—with TFCC repair to improve pain relief [24] and to provide successful treatment of persistent ulnar wrist pain following TFCC debridement [6]. Most recently Minami and Kato have reported successful treatment of TFCC tears associated with positive ulnar variance using ulnar shortening osteotomy alone [25].

The use of the pronated-grip radiograph therefore attempts to image the dynamic increase in ulnar variance that may accompany forceful grip and pronation. Friedman and colleagues have reported that a maximum grip effort resulted in an average increase in ulnar variance of 1.95 mm in asymptomatic volunteers [5]. Tomaino showed an identical average increase in the measurement of ulnar variance in light of the fact that measurements in both reports were to the nearest 0.5 mm [17]. Although these two studies do not prove that ulnar recession is required when variance becomes positive on the pronated-grip radiograph, pathomechanical and pathoanatomic data suggest that such positive variance may cause a problem [1,2,11]. Indeed, high resolution MR imaging has shown that the TFCC disc is thinner during forearm pronation [26], and it is known that the undersurface of the TFCC is innervated [12] and undergoes degeneration before perforation [11].

Although MR imaging may reveal marrow edema in the ulnar corner of the lunate, TFCC perforation, ulnar chondrosis, and a tear of the LT ligament [27,28] (Fig. 3), the authors no longer routinely order an MRI if the clinical suspicion is high for ulnar impaction and when variance is positive on a pronated-grip radiograph.

Treatment

When the history lacks a discrete traumatic precipitant for pain in the presence of a suggestive

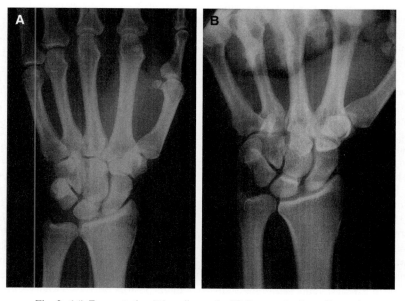

Fig. 2. (*A*) Zero rotation PA radiograph. (*B*) Pronated grip radiograph.

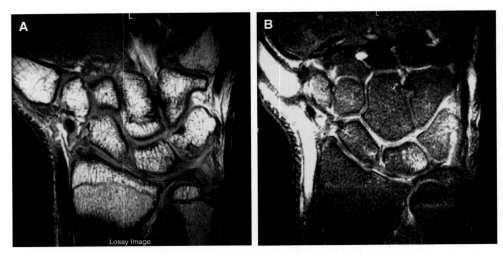

Fig. 3. (A) T-1. (B) MR images show lunate marrow edema.

examination, as described previously, and when ulnar variance is positive on a neutral rotation radiograph, the authors hypothesize that a class II lesion is present. When a neutral rotation radiograph demonstrates neutral or negative ulnar variance but the pronated-grip view demonstrates positive ulnar variance, the authors have found that a positive ulnar stress test in combination with a tender fovea correlate highly with a positive finding at the time of wrist arthroscopy. The authors routinely perform a corticosteroid injection into the ulnocarpal joint at presentation. This frequently provides transient relief of symptoms, at least, but not always.

For degenerative TFCC tears, ulnar recession with ulnar-shortening osteotomy or open wafer resection commonly provides satisfactory pain relief without the need for concomitant debridement of associated TFCC or LT tears. Indeed, even post-traumatic perforations of the TFCC have been treated with ulnar recession [29] or by partial excision [30]. Nevertheless, incomplete pain relief has been reported following debridement alone in as many as 25% of wrists, regardless of whether the tear is post-traumatic or degenerative, but only recently have the potential implications of positive ulnar variance been considered [17,23,25]. Although complete distal ulna excision (Darrach procedure) is an option when DRUJ arthritis accompanies ulnar impaction syndrome, it should be avoided for ulnar impaction alone, except perhaps in low-demand wrists, because loss of grip strength and radioulnar impingement may result [31].

The authors address two open treatment options, ulnar shortening osteotomy [1,2,32,33] and the wafer procedure [10,13,34–36], and the authors' current preference, arthroscopic wafer distal ulna resection [8,37].

Ulnar shortening osteotomy

Although ulnar-shortening osteotomy [1,2,32, 33] has been the standard procedure for ulnar impaction syndrome and recently has been advocated in wrists with neutral and negative variance also [33], the potential for hardware complications and nonunion are not insignificant [34]. When a prominent ulnar styloid accompanies positive variance and stylocarpal impaction [7,38], the authors selectively perform ulnar shortening (Fig. 4).

Open wafer procedure

The wafer procedure is an attractive alternative to ulnar shortening osteotomy in wrists with painful impaction, because it avoids risk for nonunion and hardware-related complications [34,36] (Fig. 5). Tomaino and Shah reported a retrospective evaluation of the wafer procedure that showed that it was successful [36]. With the exception of one patient who required distal ulna excision but who continued to complain of pain at final follow-up nevertheless, a provocative ulnar stress test failed to elicit symptoms in 25 of 26 patients postoperatively. Twenty-three of 26 patients (88%) were completely satisfied with their wrist

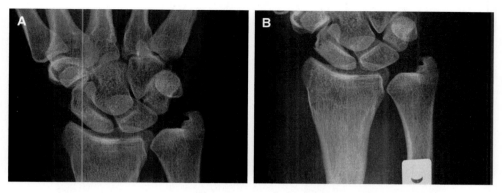

Fig. 4. (*A*) PA radiograph shows positive ulnar variance and a prominent ulnar styloid process. (*B*) Ulnar shortening osteotomy leveled the ulna and avoided the risk for subsequent pain from ongoing stylocarpal impaction.

postoperatively. They noted that pain relief typically occurred by 10–12 weeks after surgery, but most patients appreciated improvement as early as 6 weeks.

Feldon and colleagues originally suggested that greater than 4 mm of positive ulnar variance contraindicated wafer excision [13]. No patient in the series reported by Tomaino and Shah had resection greater than 4 mm; hence, their data neither refuted nor supported Feldon's original caution. The authors believe that the prominence of the ulnar styloid process and the potential for stylocarpal impaction [7,38] contraindicates use of wafer resection but do not regard the measurement of ulnar variance itself as an absolute contraindication.

In light of the potential for poor outcome following debridement of traumatic and degenerative tears in which ulnar variance is positive [23] and the observation that dynamic increases in ulnar variance in wrists with short or level ulnas may accompany pronation and grip [5,16], the authors routinely use the measurement of variance taken from a pronated grip radiograph to plan the thickness of the wafer to be resected. This ensures that adequate ulnocarpal decompression is afforded despite dynamic changes in ulnar length that may accompany forceful grip and forearm pronation. Even when the width of the resected wafer is planned based on the pronated-grip radiograph and is performed after accurate intraoperative measurement with a ruler, the authors have observed that postoperative neutral-rotation radiographs frequently show less resection than expected. Postoperative pronated-grip radiographs often provide a more accurate picture of the amount of wafer resected.

At the time of wafer resection the authors carefully draw a line across the distal ulna at the level of the osteotomy and then inspect the cartilage of the ulnar seat to ensure that at least 50% remains to articulate with the sigmoid notch. The authors have not been forced to decrease the magnitude of the wafer resection to comply with this guideline in any of the cases in this study but would not hesitate to remove a slightly narrower wafer if required.

The authors remain confident about the efficacy of an open wafer procedure as an alternative to ulnar shortening osteotomy for treatment of ulnar impaction syndrome but have elected arthroscopic wafer resection, as described below, since 1998.

Arthroscopic wafer procedure

Because TFCC debridement alone may not provide complete pain relief in wrists with positive ulnar variance, and in light of the efficacy of wafer distal ulna resection as treatment for ulnar impaction syndrome [10,13,35,36] and the biomechanical effect of an arthroscopic wafer procedure in unloading the ulnocarpal joint [14], Tomaino and Weiser evaluated the efficacy of an arthroscopic wafer procedure and TFCC debridement as treatment for post-traumatic and degenerative TFCC tears associated with positive ulnar variance [8]. Wafer resection was performed through the TFCC perforation using the 3-4 and 6R portals. Intraoperative radiographs were not taken; rather, a 2.9-mm burr was used as a guide regarding the amount of ulna to resect relative to the height of the lunate fossa cartilage (Fig. 6).

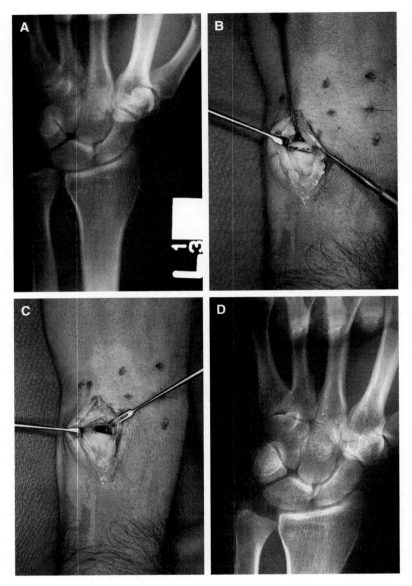

Fig. 5. (*A*) Preoperative pronated grip radiograph. (*B*) Intraoperative picture before and (*C*) after wafer resection. (*D*) Postoperative grip radiograph.

At final review nine patients were very satisfied and three were satisfied. Among the former group, complete resolution of pain occurred in eight; one rated pain as minimal. Among the three patients who were only satisfied with the procedure, one had no pain but complained of portal sensitivity ulnarly, one complained of minimal pain referable to the scapholunate joint, and one had minimal ulnar wrist pain during gripping activities [8].

The ulnocarpal stress test failed to elicit pain in any patient, and the postoperative pronated-grip radiograph revealed that ulnar variance was neutral in all wrists.

The appreciation of class II A and B lesions (TFCC wear and lunate chondrosis) at the time of the arthroscopic evaluation has allowed confirmation of the diagnosis of early stages of ulnar impaction. TFCC thinning and pitting is

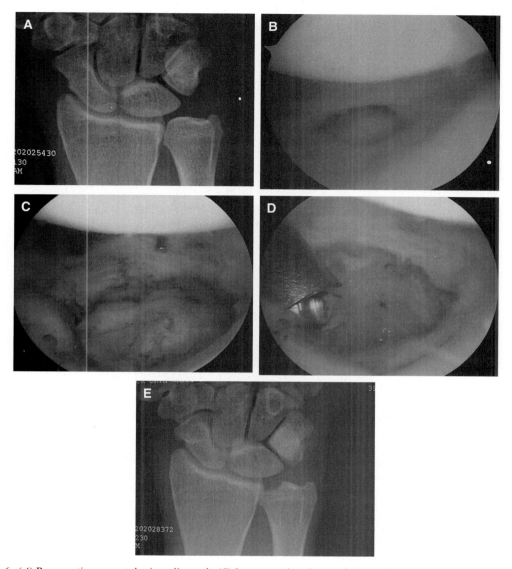

Fig. 6. (*A*) Preoperative pronated grip radiograph. (*B*) Intraoperative picture of class II C TFCC tear. (*C*) After TFCC debridement. (*D*) After wafer resection. (*E*) Postoperative grip radiograph.

noted easily. Because of favorable results of arthroscopic wafer resection in the setting of TFCC perforation [8] and the knowledge that isolated TFCC disc excision decreases ulnocarpal load and may address painful undersurface fibrillation [11,12], the authors have been evaluating prospectively the results of arthroscopic TFCC disc excision and wafer resection for class II A and B ulnar impaction for more than 2 years. Inclusion criteria have included TFCC wear without

perforation and positive ulnar variance on the zero-rotation or pronated-grip radiograph. The volar and dorsal radioulnar ligaments and the attachment of the TFCC to the ulnar styloid are preserved (Fig. 7). A wafer resection then is performed as described by Tomaino and Weiser [8]. Fourteen of 16 patients have experienced satisfactory pain relief. The authors are awaiting a minimum follow-up of 1 year for all patients before publishing this series but are continuing to pursue

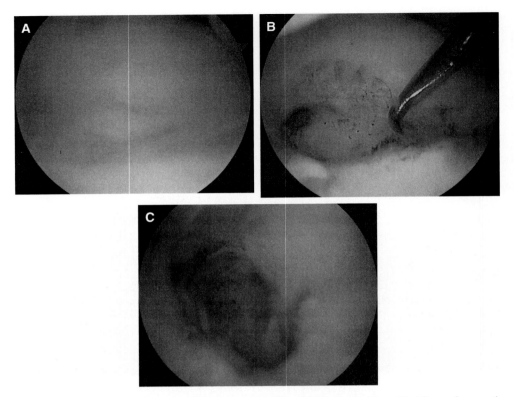

Fig. 7. (*A*) Intraoperative picture shows TFCC wear. (*B*) After TFCC disc excision. (*C*) After wafer resection.

this alternative to open wafer or ulnar shortening osteotomy in patients who have early stages of ulnar impaction syndrome.

Summary

Although Palmer's classification of TFCC lesions differentiates post-traumatic central perforations (IA tears) from degenerative tears secondary to ulnocarpal impaction (IIC) [3], the distinction is not always clear clinically. In the final analysis, the literature suggests that as many as 25% of wrists with TFCC tears have residual symptoms following arthroscopic debridement alone [23], and it is likely that static or dynamic ulnar positive variance plays a role [2,5,17,25]. The authors' results suggest that combined arthroscopic TFCC debridement and wafer resection are feasible and efficacious as treatment for all stages of ulnar impaction syndrome. When class II A and B changes are observed, that is, when a TFCC perforation has not yet developed, the authors have observed favorable results in most patients following arthroscopic TFCC central disc excision and wafer resection as an alternative to ulnar shortening osteotomy [33] or open wafer excision [10].

References

[1] Chun S, Palmer AK. The ulnar impaction syndrome: follow-up of ulnar shortening osteotomy. J Hand Surg Am 1993;18:46–53.

[2] Friedman SL, Palmer AK. The ulnar impaction syndrome. Hand Clinics 1991;7(2):295–320.

[3] Palmer AK. Triangular fibrocartilage complex lesions: a classification. J Hand Surg Am 1989;14: 594–606.

[4] Palmer AK, Werner FW. Biomechanics of the distal radioulnar joint. Clin Orthop 1984;187:26–35.

[5] Friedman SL, Palmer AK, Short WH, et al. The change in ulnar variance with grip. J Hand Surg Am 1993;18:713–6.

[6] Hulsizer D, Weiss AC, Akelman E. Ulna-shortening osteotomy after failed arthroscopic debridement of

the triangular fibrocartilage complex. J Hand Surg Am 1997;22:694–8.

[7] Tomaino MM, Towers JD, Gainer M. Carpal impaction with the ulnar styloid process: treatment with partial resection. J Hand Surg Br 2001;26: 252–5.

[8] Tomaino MM, Weiser RW. Combined arthroscopic TFCC debridement and wafer resection of the distal ulna in wrists with triangular fibrocartilage complex tears and positive ulnar variance. J Hand Surg Am 2000;26:1047–52.

[9] Palmer AK, Glisson RR, Werner FW. Relationship between ulnar variance and triangular fibrocartilage complex thickness. J Hand Surg [Am] 1984;9:681–3.

[10] Tomaino MM. Results of the wafer procedure in ulnar impaction syndrome in the ulnar negative and neutral wrist. J Hand Surg [Br] 1999;24:671–5.

[11] Tomaino MM. Ulnar impaction syndrome in the ulnar negative and neutral wrist. Diagnosis and pathoanatomy. J Hand Surg Br 1998;23:754–7.

[12] Ohmori M, Azuma H. Morphology and distribution of nerve endings in the human triangular fibrocartilage complex. J Hand Surg [Am] 1998; 23:522–5.

[13] Feldon P, Terrono AL, Belsky MR. Wafer distal ulna resection for triangular fibrocartilage tears and/or ulna impaction syndrome. J Hand Surg Am 1992;17:731–7.

[14] Wnorowski DC, Palmer AK, Werner FW, et al. Anatomic and biomechanical analysis of the arthroscopic wafer procedure. Arthroscopy 1992;8: 204–12.

[15] Markolf KL, Tejwani SG, Benhaim P. Effects of wafer resection and hemiresection from the distal ulna on load-sharing at the wrist: a cadaveric study. J Hand Surg Am 2005;30:351–8.

[16] Tomaino MM, Rubin DA. The value of the pronated grip view radiograph in assessing dynamic ulnar positive variance: a case report. Am J Orthop 1999;3:180–1.

[17] Tomaino MM. The importance of the pronated grip x-ray. J Hand Surg Am 2000;25:352–7.

[18] Ekenstam FW, Palmer AK, Glisson RR. The load on the radius and ulna in different positions of the wrist and forearm. A cadaver study. Acta Orthop Scand 1984;55(3):363–5.

[19] Pfaeffle HJ, Manson T, Fischer KJ, et al. Axial loading alters ulnar variance and distal ulna load with forearm pronation. Pittsburgh Orthop J 1999;10: 101–2.

[20] Palmer AK, Glisson RR, Werner FW. Ulnar variance determination. J Hand Surg 1982;7:376–9.

[21] Nakamura R, Horii E, Imaeda T, et al. The ulnocarpal stress test in the diagnosis of ulnar-sided wrist pain. J Hand Surg Br 1997;22:719–23.

[22] Steyers CM, Blair WF. Measuring ulnar variance: a comparison of techniques. J Hand Surg Am 1989; 14:607–12.

[23] Minami A, Ishikawa J, Suenage N, et al. Clinical results of treatment of triangular fibrocartilage complex tears by arthroscopic debridement. J Hand Surg Am 1996;21:406–11.

[24] Trumble TE, Gilbert M, Vedder N. Ulnar shortening combined with arthroscopic repairs in the delayed management of triangular fibrocartilage complex tears. J Hand Surg Am 1997;22:807–13.

[25] Minami K, Kato H. Ulnar shortening for triangular fibrocartilage complex tears associated with ulnar positive variance. J Hand Surg Am 1998;23:904–8.

[26] Nakamura T, Yabe Y, Horiuchi Y. Dynamic changes in the shape of the triangular fibrocartilage complex during rotation demonstrated with high resolution magnetic resonance imaging. J Hand Surg Br 1999;24:338–41.

[27] Escobedo EM, Bergman G, Hunter JC. MR imaging of ulnar impaction. Skeletal Radiol 1993;24:85–90.

[28] Imaeda T, Nakamura R, Shionoya K, et al. Ulnar impaction syndrome: MR imaging findings. Radiology 1996;201:495–500.

[29] Boulas JH, Milek MA. Ulnar shortening for tears of the triangular fibrocartilaginous complex. J Hand Surg Am 1990;15:415–20.

[30] Menon J, Wood VE, Schoene HR. Isolated tears of the triangular fibrocartilage of the wrist; results of partial excision. J Hand Surg Am 1984;9:527–30.

[31] Bieber EJ, Linscheid RL, Dobyns JH, et al. Failed distal ulna resection. J Hand Surg Am 1988;13: 193–200.

[32] Loh YC, Van Den Abbellek, Stanley JK, et al. The results of ulnar shortening for ulnar impaction syndrome. J Hand Surg Br 1999;24:316–20.

[33] Tatebe M, Nakamura R, Horii E, et al. Results of ulnar shortening osteotomy for ulnocarpal impaction syndrome in wrists with neutral or negative ulnar variance. J Hand Surg Br 2005;30:129–32.

[34] Constantine KJ, Tomaino MM, Herndon JH, et al. Comparison of ulnar shortening osteotomy and the wafer procedure for ulnar impaction syndrome. J Hand Surg Am 2000;25:55–60.

[35] Schuurman AH, Bos KE. The ulno-carpal abutment syndrome. J Hand Surg Br 1995;20:171–7.

[36] Tomaino MM, Shah M. Treatment of ulnar impaction syndrome with the wafer procedure. Am J Ortho 2001;30:129–33.

[37] Osterman AL. Arthroscopic debridement of triangular fibrocartilage complex tears. Arthroscopy 1990;6:120–4.

[38] Topper SM, Wood MB, Ruby LK. Ulnar styloid impaction syndrome. J Hand Surg Am 1997;22: 699–704.

Hand Clin 21 (2005) 577–589

Management of the Distal Radioulnar Joint in Rheumatoid Arthritis

Steve K. Lee, MD*, Michael R. Hausman, MD

*Hand and Upper Extremity Service, Department of Orthopaedic Surgery,
The Mount Sinai School of Medicine, 5 East 98th Street,
Box 1188, New York, NY 10029, USA*

Most patients (80%) who have rheumatoid arthritis (RA) manifest signs and symptoms in the wrist [1]. Wrist dysfunction is a potential source of major disability, because the wrist places the hand in positions of optimal function and has been called the keystone of the hand [2–4]. Rheumatoid disease can affect all three major articulations of the wrist: the distal radioulnar joint (DRUJ), the radiocarpal joint, and the midcarpal joint [5]. Of these, the DRUJ is the most commonly involved [6]. Unfortunately the DRUJ is particularly susceptible to the ravages of RA.

Because of the mismatched radius of curvature of the larger sigmoid notch of the distal radius and the smaller ulnar head, the DRUJ is inherently unstable, with only approximately 20% of DRUJ stability attributed to its articular contact [7,8]. Synovial-lined ligamentous stabilizers are therefore critical to DRUJ stability, yet uniquely vulnerable to rheumatoid disease [5,9,10]. Rheumatoid synovial hypertrophy, with its resultant inflammatory enzymes, leads to ligamentous attenuation and joint erosion [5].

In the rheumatoid wrist, static *and* dynamic stabilizers are altered by the rheumatoid process. Static stabilizers include bone and ligaments; dynamic stabilizers are muscle-tendon units. The bony stabilizers of the distal ulna and distal radius

are eroded by rheumatoid synovitis. Erosion of the dorsal border of the sigmoid notch of the radius is associated with DRUJ subluxation and significant alteration of DRUJ kinematics [11]. The primary ligamentous stabilizing unit of the DRUJ, the TFCC complex [9], is usually attenuated or destroyed [12,13].

The extensor carpi ulnaris (ECU) is one of the most important dynamic stabilizers of the wrist [13,14]. Elucidated in EMG studies, the ECU contracts during dorsiflexion and co-contracts during palmar flexion [13]. In the rheumatoid wrist, the ECU tendon compartment is destroyed and the tendon dislocates in a palmar direction, destabilizing the DRUJ and radiocarpal joints. In the abnormal palmarly dislocated position of the ECU, there is no ECU co-contraction during palmar flexion, demonstrating its loss of ability to dynamically stabilize the DRUJ. ECU co-contraction returns after it is reduced back to its normal dorsal position [13]. Furthermore, in pronation, the ECU depresses the ulnar head, stabilizing the DRUJ.

Clinical presentation

In 1963, Swedish hand surgeon Magnus Backdahl coined the term caput ulnae syndrome in his classic monograph about the pathologic changes of the DRUJ in RA [13] (Fig. 1). The pathoanatomic changes include palmar subluxation and supination of the carpus (with the appearance of a dorsally prominent ulnar head), palmar dislocation of the ECU tendon, and possible carpal translocation [3]. Approximately one third of patients with RA develop caput ulnae syndrome

No benefits in any form have been received or will be received from a commercial party related directly or indirectly to the subject of this article.

* Corresponding author.

E-mail address: steve.lee@msnyuhealth.org (S.K. Lee).

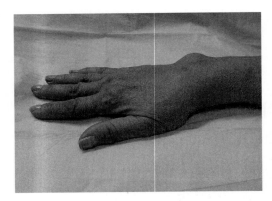

Fig. 1. Caput ulnae syndrome with prominent ulnar head.

[1,4]. Clinically the syndrome presents as follows [13]:

1. Pain and weakness with range of motion, especially with forearm rotation; loss of range of motion, particularly in supination [1]
2. A prominent bump on the dorsal ulnar aspect of the wrist (caput ulnae) capable of abnormal dorsopalmar displacement (piano-key sign), often with painful crepitus
3. Soft swelling on the ulnar dorsal aspect of the wrist and hand, with the extensor retinaculum forming a depression across it
4. Potential finger extensor tendon ruptures with one or several ulnar fingers dropped (Vaughan-Jackson syndrome) [15,16]

Although Vaughan-Jackson [15,16] and others [17] originally attributed tendon ruptures to abrasion or attrition over bony prominences, the true cause is multifactorial, with direct synovial invasion [17,18] and degeneration coupled with devascularization and loss of nutrition playing large roles [1,19,20] (Fig. 2).

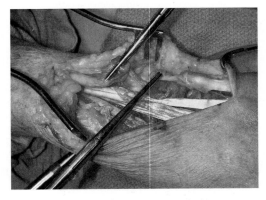

Fig. 2. Vaughan-Jackson syndrome of ulnar extensor tendon ruptures.

It is paramount to assess how much of the patient's symptoms are originating from the nearby joints, most notably the radiocarpal, midcarpal, and metacarpophalangeal joints. Determining how much pain is present with wrist flexion and extension versus forearm rotation is key in the assessment. Also important to the evaluation of forearm rotation is the proximal radioulnar joint (PRUJ) of the elbow. Berger emphasizes that the forearm is a bicondylar joint articulating through the PRUJ and DRUJ [21].

Diagnostic imaging

Radiographs

Standard posteroanterior, oblique, and lateral radiographs should be obtained and critically evaluated for the DRUJ and surrounding joints. In a longitudinal radiographic analysis of RA in the hand and wrist, the DRUJ had the highest percentage of early (31%) and late (75%) involvement of all studied wrist and hand joints [6] (Fig. 3A,B). The most common wrist deformity on late films was ulnar translocation of the carpus [6]. The DRUJ displays a typical pattern of bony destruction: erosions of the inferior portion of the DRUJ, the prestyloid recess, and the ECU subsheath [1]. Of particular interest is Freiberg and Weinstein's scallop sign, in which the sigmoid notch of the distal radius has an erosive scalloped out concavity that correlates with spontaneous extensor tendon ruptures [22] (Fig. 4). Other modalities such as computed tomography or magnetic resonance imaging usually are not necessary in the evaluation of RA in the DRUJ.

Treatment

Nonoperative treatment

Treatment of RA is by a multidisciplinary team approach. Rheumatologists, physical, hand, and occupational therapists, and orthopedic and hand surgeons comprise the team. Investigators have found that rheumatologists and hand surgeons differ in their assessment as to the efficacy of hand surgery [23]. Despite these differences, collaboration between these two physician groups should be fostered and is undoubtedly beneficial to the patient. Nonoperative treatment consists of hand and occupational therapy, orthotic splinting, and pharmacologic agents managed by a rheumatologist [1,2,24]. Hand and occupational therapy consists of exercise and activity training to optimize independent function.

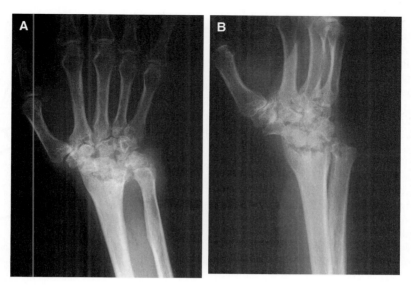

Fig. 3. (*A*) Posteroanterior wrist radiograph demonstrating severe osseous destruction of rheumatoid arthritis. (*B*) Oblique wrist radiograph demonstrating caput ulnae syndrome.

Static wrist splinting in neutral should help reduce inflammation, support unstable joints, decrease deformity, and improve function [1,18,24]. Disease modifying antirheumatic drugs (DMARDs), such as methotrexate, leflunomide, etanercept, and infliximab, decrease the rheumatoid synovial proliferation and joint and soft tissue destruction [5]. Because of their potential effect on already weakened tendons, corticosteroid injections in the DRUJ region are not recommended [1,24].

Operative treatment

As stated by Vaughan-Jackson, "For in rheumatoid arthritis one deformity leads to another and early attention is essential" [13]. When unacceptable pain, dysfunction, and deformity exist despite appropriate nonoperative management, surgery may be indicated. Deformity alone is not necessarily an indication for surgery if the patient is functional and does not have significant pain [24]. Although the time frame is controversial, most investigators recommend 4–6 months of appropriate nonoperative treatment before considering surgery [1,18,24] unless tendon rupture has already occurred, in which case surgery should proceed expeditiously to prevent further ruptures [17–19,24]. Goals in surgical treatment are (1) pain relief, (2) preservation or restoration of function [2], (3) prevention of further destruction [2], and (4) cosmesis [1]. Cosmesis historically has been listed as the least important of surgical goals

for RA. A recent study, however, demonstrated the importance of cosmesis to patient satisfaction. Mandl and colleagues found that the strongest determinant of patient satisfaction was postoperative hand appearance [25]. In general, surgical outcomes are best when performed before the patient displays severe joint destruction, fixed contractures, subluxation, or dislocation [3].

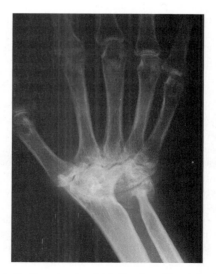

Fig. 4. Scallop sign in which the sigmoid notch of the distal radius has an erosive scalloped out concavity that correlates with spontaneous extensor tendon ruptures.

The surgical approach

A dorsal midline incision is made to the level of the extensor retinaculum, preserving longitudinal veins and cutaneous nerves. Linear incisions and careful hemostasis are important to avoid postoperative wound or skin complications [1]. The retinaculum is raised from the radial and ulnar aspects, maintaining the ulnar aspect of the extensor compartment of the extensor digiti minimi (EDM) as its base as described by Spinner and Kaplan [14] (Fig. 5). The radial and ulnar retinacular flaps are raised like wings with a central base. The radial flaps are divided in half; the proximal half is used as a sling around the ECU tendon to maintain it in its dorsal, reduced, stabilizing position. The distal radial half of the extensor retinaculum is repaired back into its original position after tenosynovectomy is performed. The ulnar flap is used to reconstruct the dorsal DRUJ capsule (Fig. 6).

If a debridement of the DRUJ without a distal ulna bony procedure is planned, the dorsal radioulnar ligament must be preserved while the DRUJ is approached. This is performed by making an L-shaped incision with the long arm in line with the ulnar aspect of the radius and the short arm just proximal to the dorsal radioulnar ligament, which is 4–5 mm wide at the distal dorsal ulnar corner of the radius and has a deep attachment on the ulnar fovea and a superficial attachment at the base of the ulnar styloid. For added pain relief, a posterior interosseous neurectomy of 1 cm as described by Buck-Gramcko [26] is recommended [1]. The posterior interosseous nerve lies in the radial aspect of the floor of the fourth dorsal extensor compartment.

Synovectomy, tenosynovectomy

DRUJ synovectomy and extensor tendon tenosynovectomy are usually part of any operation involving the DRUJ. In the rare patient who presents with persistent symptomatic rheumatoid synovitis and tenosynovitis with little or no radiographic evidence of joint pathology [1], synovectomy or tenosynovectomy alone may be indicated [5,24]. The usual patient who has RA, however, presents with more advanced disease requiring soft tissue rebalancing and osseous procedures. The usual late presentation of patients who have RA may be because of differing opinions between hand surgeons and rheumatologists regarding efficacy of operative procedures. Alderman and colleagues reported that 93% of hand surgeons believed that prophylactic extensor

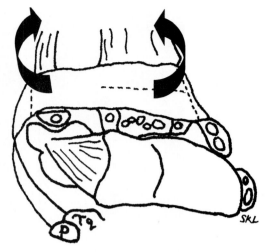

Fig. 5. Incisions on the extensor retinaculum. The base of the radial and ulnar halves is the ulnar aspect of the extensor digiti minimi dorsal compartment.

tenosynovectomy prevented extensor tendon rupture, whereas only 53% of rheumatologists agreed [23]. Certainly the role of synovectomy and tenosynovectomy early in the disease process needs to be better defined [5]. Nevertheless, if a patient does have a procedure for RA in the wrist, synovectomy and tenosynovectomy is an integral part of any operation. During tenosynovectomy, hypertrophic synovium is excised systematically from each dorsal compartment. Tendons at risk

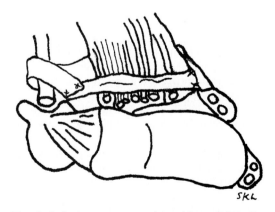

Fig. 6. Soft tissue reconstruction with an ECU sling from the proximal radial half of the extensor retinaculum. The distal radial half of the retinaculum is repaired over the extensor tendons. The ulnar half of the retinaculum is repaired palmar to the ECU tendon to augment the capsular repair.

for rupture are sutured to adjacent intact tendons proximally and distally to the attenuated site [3]. Clayton reported that up to 6 years after dorsal tenosynovectomy, patients did not have recurrence of rheumatoid tenosynovitis and no tendons had ruptured even though some were frayed at the time of surgery [17]. Millender and colleagues support early tenosynovectomy in patients who have (1) persistent dorsal tenosynovitis despite adequate medical treatment, (2) extensor tendon rupture, or (3) recurrent dorsal tenosynovitis; they reported low recurrence of tenosynovitis and low postoperative extensor tendon rupture rates [18]. Clawson and Stern support synovectomy, stating that although recurrence may occur, recurrent synovitis is generally less severe [1].

Reconstruction for tendon rupture

Tendon rupture is often insidious and not associated with trauma, strenuous exercise, or significant pain. As stated by Moore and colleagues, "early aggressive treatment of distal radioulnar joint derangements in the rheumatoid wrist is recommended to forestall many cases of tendon rupture" [19]. If a patient who has RA presents with tendon rupture, surgical intervention should proceed urgently to halt progression of more tendon ruptures [17–19,24]. The results of tendon reconstruction after rupture are inferior to the function of intact tendons saved from rupture by prophylactic tenosynovectomy [17].

If a patient presents with tendon rupture, direct repair is usually impossible because of retraction, shortening and fibrosis of muscle, and destruction of remaining tendon from direct invasion of rheumatoid synovium [18]. Tendon transfer is usually necessary to restore function. This usually is performed in conjunction with procedures to the DRUJ, as discussed subsequently. The most commonly ruptured tendons in descending order are EDM [19], extensor digitorum communis (EDC) to the small [18] and ring [19] fingers in approximately equal amounts, EDC to the middle finger, extensor pollicis longus (EPL), EDC to the index, extensor indicis proprius (EIP), extensor carpi radialis longus (ECRL) and brevis (ECRB) [19,20,27], and uncommonly, extensor carpi ulnaris (ECU) [28].

Reports of extensor tendon reconstruction vary in technique, but fortunately most report good results with several different transfers, presumably because of the low demand of the patient who has RA and the tenodesis effect aiding in extensor tendon transfers. The procedures performed most commonly are end-to-side tendon transfer [29,30] and EIP transfers [28,30]. For EPL rupture, EIP transfer was performed most commonly [18,19].

Millender and colleagues recommended end-to-side adjacent transfer for small finger extensor tendon rupture if the distal end was long enough; otherwise an EIP transfer was used. For double rupture of ring and small fingers, they recommended EIP to the small finger and end-to-side of the ring to the intact middle finger tendon. For multiple ruptures, a combination of EIP transfer and end-to-side transfers were considered if possible; otherwise, FDS or wrist extensor (ECRL) tendon transfer was used. The excursion of a wrist extensor is less than the finger extensor; there will always be incomplete MCP joint motion, but the tenodesis effect aids in making an acceptable result as long as the wrist has adequate motion [18].

Clayton reported that there is no significant difference between distant tendon transfer and adjacent end-to-side transfer and that the simplest procedure is probably the best. For multiple ruptures, he reported that single wrist extensor to EDCs of middle, ring, and small fingers gave good results [17].

Moore and colleagues reported that for ruptures of the small or ring fingers, or small and ring fingers, good results were obtained by end-to-side transfer to the intact EDC of the middle finger. Cases of multiple tendon ruptures were treated with FDS from the ring or middle fingers through a window in the interosseous membrane at a point just proximal to the pronator quadratus [19] or around the subcutaneous border of the radius [31]. They reported no difference in outcome between the two FDS routing techniques. FDS transfers performed best in patients who had good wrist motion and no metacarpophalangeal (MCP) disease. Several advantages of FDS transfer include exceptional length of tendon transfer, adequate amplitude and strength, lack of morbidity, and ease of harvest. Postoperative extensor lag was common; therefore, erring on the side of increased tension of the transfer is recommended.

The authors' preferred method is to treat with the simplest approach possible, which is usually end-to-side transfers to adjacent intact EDC tendons and the use of the EIP or ECRL transfer for greater than two ruptures or short distal tendon stumps. Postoperatively the wrist and fingers are immobilized for 4 weeks with the wrist extended 20°, MCP joints flexed 20°, and IPs at 0°. At 4 weeks a dynamic splint is fabricated and gentle passive range of motion started. Support is used for 6–8 weeks.

Distal radioulnar joint osseous procedures

When there is derangement of the articular surfaces of the DRUJ with pain or limitation of motion, DRUJ osseous procedures are indicated. The major categories and subcategories include (1) distal ulnar resection, either (a) transverse (Darrach) [32–34] or (b) oblique, (i) hemi-resection interposition [35] or (ii) matched distal ulnar resection [36]; (2) DRUJ fusion with proximal ulnar pseudarthrosis (Sauve-Kapandji) [37]; and (3) distal ulnar prosthesis [38]. Which procedure is best is controversial. The two procedures used most commonly are the transverse distal ulna resection with soft tissue reconstruction (modified Darrach) and the DRUJ fusion with proximal ulnar pseudarthrosis (modified Sauve-Kapandji). Understandably many investigators have attempted to discard eponyms, because the procedures most surgeons perform today are modifications from the operations originally described. Despite these well meaning attempts, the eponyms seem to have prevailed in hand surgery vocabulary; the authors therefore refer to such procedures as "Darrach" and "Sauve-Kapandji," with the understanding that the current operations are modifications, as we describe.

Transverse distal ulna resection (Darrach)

According to Goldfarb and Stern, caput ulnae syndrome is treated most commonly with the Darrach procedure [5]. The Darrach has the longest track record of the two bony procedures most widely accepted. Although Severinus was the first to report resection of the distal ulna in 1644 [39], Darrach popularized the procedure that still bears his name [32,33]. Darrach's original indication was for traumatic anterior dislocation of the head of the ulna [32]; Smith-Peterson and colleagues were the first to report its use in patients who have RA [40].

There are many reports that support the Darrach procedure for patients who have RA [5,12,24,29,30,41], and most demonstrate good results with 60%–95% pain relief and less than 10% ulnar stump pain or recurrence of DRUJ synovitis [24]. Rana and Taylor reported 93% pain relief and 87% with full rotation in a series of 86 wrists [29]. Most investigators also report no extensor tendon ruptures postoperatively [12,29,42]. Excessive resection and poor soft tissue repair has been associated with extensor tendon rupture [43].

When assessing the results of the Darrach, it is important to separate the patients who have RA from the patients who have post-traumatic arthrosis. Fraser and colleagues compared the Darrach procedure in the two groups and found that 86% of patients who had RA were satisfied with the Darrach, whereas only 36% of patients who had post-traumatic arthrosis were satisfied [44].

The Darrach procedure has undergone many modifications. In the original description, "the lower inch of the ulna was removed subperiosteally," "leaving the ulnar styloid intact" [32,33]. Dingman reported that whether the procedure was performed subperiosteally or extraperiosteally or whether the ulnar styloid was excised or left in situ made no difference in the results. What did make a difference was how much bone was resected. The best results occurred when the minimal amount was resected, just to the level of the sigmoid notch [12,29,34]. Leaving attachments of the important dynamic stabilizer, the pronator quadratus, to the ulnar stump improves outcome.

Regarding ulnar translocation, reports vary. Rana and Taylor reported that 10% of patients had ulnar translocation after the Darrach procedure, but in no case did this affect the clinical results [29]. Cracchiolo and Marmor reported no translocation postoperatively in 42 wrists [12]. Posner and Ambrose stated that "ulnar head resection in the presence of damage to the extrinsic wrist ligaments may exacerbate a carpal shift, but it will not, in the absence of damage to these ligaments, cause a shift" [41]. Van Gemert and Spauwen concluded that ulnar translocation more often is caused by the rheumatoid process itself than by distal ulna resection [45]. Melone and Taras reported that 4 of 50 (8%) went on to excessive, disabling ulnar translocation [30]. Thirupathi reported on 38 wrists followed for 5–14 years, with an average follow-up of 7.4 years. Forty-four percent displayed carpal translocation with progression occurring in a linear fashion with the years of follow-up [20]. Unfortunately most of these reports do not specify preoperative criteria, such as pre-existing ulnar translocation, palmar subluxation, excessive radial inclination, or quality of distal radial ulnar bone stock, all of which are important parameters that influence the risk for postoperative translocation.

Darrach—indications

1. Older, sedentary patient with no pre-existing radiocarpal instability (see section on contraindications)

2. Radiocarpal joint stabilized by pseudarthrosis, ulnar shelf, or auto-fusion; in these cases, ulnar translocation does not progress [30,46,47]
3. Inadequate distal ulnar bone stock for Sauve-Kapandji

Darrach—contraindications
1. Pre-existing radiocarpal instability [41] or tendency as heralded by:
   a. Ulnar translocation; the most practical and best method to determine ulnar translocation [48] is to evaluate whether there is more than 50% lunate overhang ulnar to the lunate fossa of the distal radius [30]
   b. Palmar subluxation
   c. Excessive radial inclination > 23°; these patients are susceptible to ulnar translocation [24,49,50]
   d. Excessive bone deficiency of the ulnar aspect of the distal radius; Black and colleagues reported that this predisposed the wrist to ulnar translocation [46]

If there is pre-existing radiocarpal instability, the Darrach procedure still may be performed if the carpus is stabilized concomitantly with partial (radiolunate [51] or radioscapholunate) or total wrist arthrodesis [24,52].

2. Young (< 45 years of age), active patient; although not studied specifically in patients who had RA, Bieber and colleagues reported worse results with the Darrach procedure in patients younger than 45 years of age, especially those with ligamentous laxity [53]

Darrach resection—surgical procedure and supported technical recommendations. The initial surgical approach was described previously. After the ulnar retinacular flap is raised, the DRUJ capsule is incised longitudinally just ulnar to the fifth dorsal compartment septum. The capsule and periosteum frequently is invaded with rheumatoid synovitis; synovectomy is performed. The distal ulna is osteotomized with a microsagittal saw just proximal to the sigmoid notch and is excised (Fig. 7). Resection should be limited to ≤2 cm [4,12,43,47,54]. Rana and Taylor reported distal stump clicking if more than 3.5 cm was excised and no clicking if less than 2 cm was excised [29]. Gainor and Schaberg reported that excessive resection > 2 cm may contribute to ulnar translocation [47]. It is also important to bevel the dorsal ulnar stump to decrease attritional wear on

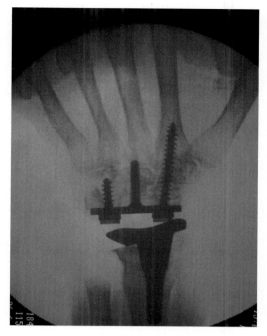

Fig. 7. Darrach distal ulna resection with total wrist arthroplasty.

overlying tendons [4]. Further synovectomy is performed once the distal ulna has been removed.

Although there are many reports of different ulnar stump stabilization techniques [1], the distally based ulnar half ECU tenodesis is used most commonly and is the authors' preferred method. A 3-mm burr is used to place a hole in the dorsal cortex of the ulnar stump and the distally based ulnar half of the ECU woven from within the ulnar canal and out the hole and sutured to itself with the ulnar stump reduced palmarly, the wrist extended 15° and ulnarly deviated 15°. The distally based ECU tenodesis increases stability and has provided good results [2,3,5,24,30,41,42,55]. Rowland and colleagues and Melone and Taras demonstrated that the ECU tenodesis corrects the wrist deformity [30,42,55]. It ulnarly deviates the radially deviated wrist and translates the carpus back radially (Fig. 8A). In the sagittal plane, the tenodesis provides a restraint to dorsopalmar instability of the ulnar stump (Fig. 8B). Leslie and colleagues reported that the distal ulna was stabilized in 96% of patients, pain was relieved in 85%, and grip strength improved in 77% [42]. Melone and Taras reported 86% of 50 wrists with highly satisfactory

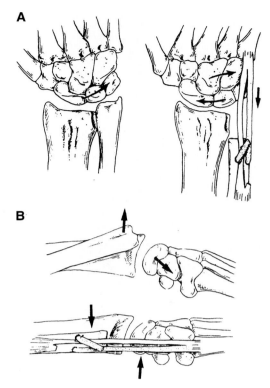

Fig. 8. (*A*) In the coronal plane, the ECU tenodesis promotes ulnar deviation and radial translation. (*B*) In the sagittal plane, the tenodesis provides a restraint to dorsopalmar instability of the ulnar stump. (*From* Melone CP Jr, Taras JS. Distal ulna resection, extensor carpi ulnaris tenodesis, and dorsal synovectomy for the rheumatoid wrist. Hand Clin 1991;7(2):335–43; with permission.)

outcome. Fourteen percent had suboptimal recovery secondary to unremitting radiocarpal disease [30]. O'Donovan and Ruby reported their series of 19 patients with distal ulnar resection and ECU tenodesis to have an average gain of 10° of prono-supination arc of motion. Wrist flexion/extension was unchanged. Eighty-five percent had complete pain relief and 15% had less pain [2]. If the ECU is not intact to use, then a distally based half FCU tenodesis may be used [41,56]. Several investigators prefer volar capsulodesis [52] or the combined ECU and FCU tenodesis [10,52,57].

Advantages of the Darrach resection
1. Predictable results, given the correct patient selection criteria is met
2. Does not rely on bony union for success

3. Able to perform on patients with inadequate bone stock of the distal ulna.

Disadvantages of the Darrach resection
1. Loss in buttress to ulnar or palmar translocation [52]
2. Possible ulnar stump instability or radioulnar convergence [52]
3. Carpal supination may be accelerated when the distal ulna is excised [24]
4. Potential rupture of extensor tendons over the ulnar stump [43]
5. Potential weakness of grip [52,53,58]

Failed Darrach resection. Failure after Darrach resection is usually from instability in the dorsopalmar plane, radioulnar convergence with resultant pain, clicking, and weakness [52], or from ulnar or palmar carpal translocation with resultant deformity and dysfunction. The failed symptomatic Darrach resection poses a difficult reconstructive surgical problem. If failure is caused by radioulnar instability or convergence, several options for treatment have been proposed. Kleinman and Greenberg recommended a distally based ECU tenodesis, pronator quadratus interposition transfer, and DRUJ pinning [59]. Breen and Jupiter reported on a combined distally based FCU tenodesis and proximally based ECU tenodesis [57]. Wolfe and colleagues have shown that wide excision of the distal ulna of 25%–50% of the ulnar length may lead to acceptable results of revision of failed distal ulna excision if the interosseous membrane is intact [60]. Creation of a one-bone forearm through radioulnar fusion or ulnar head implant arthroplasty are other options [52].

Treatment of symptomatic carpal ulnar or palmar translocation or dislocation is partial or total wrist fusion [24,51,52].

The Sauve-Kapandji procedure
Originally described by Sauve-Kapandji in 1936 [37] and erroneously credited to Lauenstein by Steindler [61], the Sauve-Kapandji (S-K) procedure is the procedure of choice for patients who have RA of the DRUJ for several investigators [38,50,62–64].

Vincent and colleagues reported dissatisfaction with their results of the Darrach resection for patients who had RA with postoperative ulnar and palmar translocation and resultant worsening of deformity and function. They reported that the S-K operation gives superior results. They commented on a particular patient who had a Darrach resection on one side and an S-K procedure on the other and had a better outcome with the S-K side. S-K prevents carpal translocation but does not arrest progression of ulnar and palmar translocation if it is present preoperatively. In this case, they recommend distal ulna resection and a wrist-stabilizing procedure, radiolunate or total wrist arthrodesis [62]. Blank and Cassidy agree that for the impending ulnocarpal translocation, radial inclination of greater than 23° or minimal radiolunate contact, S-K alone is not indicated and they recommend concomitant radiolunate or radioscapholunate fusion [24].

If there is poor distal ulna bone stock, Fujita and colleagues described making an osteotomy of the ulna 3 cm proximal to the distal end. They then make a 10-mm hole in the sigmoid notch 12–15 mm deep and pot the proximal end of the osteotomized distal ulna into this hole. It then is fixed with a cancellous bone screw. In 66 wrists, they reported 100% union, significant decrease in pain and increase in forearm rotation, and no change in carpal translation index [63].

Sauve-Kapandji—indications
1. Younger (less than 45 years of age), active patient [1]
2. Augmentation of a radiolunate fusion mass [24]

Sauve-Kapandji—contraindications
1. Pre-existing radiocarpal instability (see section on Darrach contraindications)

If there is pre-existing radiocarpal instability, S-K still may be performed if the carpus is stabilized concomitantly with partial (radiolunate [51] or radioscapholunate) or total wrist arthrodesis [4,24].

Sauve-Kapandji operation—surgical procedure and supported technical recommendations. Although originally described as approached between the ECU and FCU [37], the authors' preferred method is to approach dorsally as described in the surgical approach section. The DRUJ capsule is incised longitudinally just ulnar to the fifth dorsal compartment septum and synovectomy is performed. The DRUJ is exposed and decortication of the sigmoid notch and corresponding ulnar head is performed with a 3-mm burr. The distal ulna is reduced and two guidewires for 3.5-mm cannulated screws are placed in the distal ulna before osteotomy and destabilization of the bone. Earlier descriptions recommended 12–30 mm of

ulnar resection [50]; the authors recommend a judicious ulnar resection of 8–10 mm just proximal to the sigmoid notch to minimize ulnar stump instability and pain [52,58,65,66]. Bone graft from the resected ulnar segment then is placed in the fusion site. Preoperative ulnar positive variance should be corrected at the time of distal ulna arthrodesis [24] to slightly ulnar negative variance [52]. This may necessitate performing the osteotomy before screw fixation if the patient is ulnar positive preoperatively.

Periosteal resection and interposition of a portion of the pronator quadratus repaired to the ECU sheath should be performed to halt reconstitution of the ulna and subsequent loss of forearm rotation [50,62]. The fusion site is fixed with a cannulated 3.5-mm partially threaded screw and temporary guidewire for rotational stability. A second screw may be placed if there is adequate space on the distal ulna. It is important to arthrodese the ulnar head centered in the sigmoid notch on the anteroposterior plane and collinear to the proximal ulnar shaft (Fig. 9). Ulnar stump stabilization, particularly if the distal ulnar stump seems unstable secondary to soft tissue attenuation, should be performed. This may be done with a proximally based [67] or distally based ECU tenodesis (the authors' preferred method as described earlier in the Darrach section) or distally based FCU tenodesis [52,68].

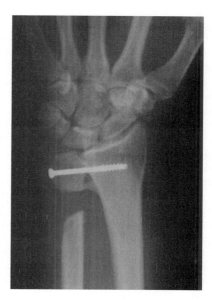

Fig. 9. Sauve-Kapandji procedure.

Advantages of the Sauve-Kapandji procedure

1. Decreases ulnar translocation and palmar subluxation if pre-existing radiocarpal instability is not present [5,47,52,65,68–71]; Vincent and colleagues reported that if translocation was present preoperatively, S-K did not stop progression; this was based on one case; in their series, no patients without translocation preoperatively developed translocation postoperatively [62]
2. Maintains a more normal load pattern between the radius and ulna, because normally 20% of axial load passes through the ulna [9]; even minor derangements in this region can result in changes of load pattern [58]
3. Retaining the ulnar head is important for the mechanism of the ECU, which adds to stability [1,58]
4. Maintains TFCC attachments [1,62]
5. Improved strength and function [1,62]

Disadvantages of the Sauve-Kapandji procedure

1. Vincent and colleagues report on a nonpainful clunk (ulnar instability) with forearm rotation in 62%, which is similar to the Darrach procedure [62]
2. Possibility of nonunion

Oblique distal ulna resection (Bowers' hemiresection-interposition versus Watson's matched distal ulnar resection)

Although these two procedures have had their proponents [35,36], few investigators currently advocate these partial resections [24]. An intact TFCC is a prerequisite for the hemiresection [35], and in patients who have RA, the triangular fibrocartilage is almost always completely destroyed [12]. Furthermore, there may be subsequent stylocarpal impingement [24].

According to Bowers and Watson, the main advantage of an oblique distal ulnar resection over a transverse resection is the preservation of the TFCC attachment and therefore increased stability of the DRUJ. Bowers presented 27 patients who had RA, all of whom had mild RA with pain but only minimal osseous destructive changes. To perform the hemiresection interposition (HIT) procedure, there must be a functionally adequate or reconstructible TFCC. If the TFCC was not reconstructible, the HIT was abandoned and a modified Darrach procedure performed. Unfortunately he did not state the percentage of patients in which this was the case [35]. Also, one can infer that for moderate to severe cases with more severe osseous destruction, a Darrach procedure was used.

Watson presented a matched distal ulnar resection that was a longer osteotomy with a broader noncontact area believed to reduce impingement problems. He presented 34 rheumatoid wrists. Thirty-three of the 34, however, also had radiocarpal fibrous nonunion or arthrodesis [36]. Although Watson presented good results, it is difficult to ascertain how beneficial the matched distal ulnar resection would be without radiocarpal fibrous nonunion or arthrodesis.

Given the problems with these reports, the paucity of new literature of their use in the patient who has RA, that most patients who have RA requiring bony procedures have incompetent TFCCs [24], and that partial resection does not allow for complete synovectomy [41], the oblique distal ulnar resections in the patient who has RA are a less favored technique.

Distal ulna prosthesis

A new concept is the replacement of the distal ulna [38,52] alone or with a sigmoid component: a total DRUJ arthroplasty. Cooney recently presented using distal ulna prostheses in three patients who had RA [38]. Although patient numbers are small, the early results are promising. To address the instability of the distal ulna, Cooney takes a sling of FCU around dorsally over the ulna and attaches it to the dorsal aspect of the radius (W. Cooney, IV, MD, personal communication, 2005). The complete topic of distal ulna prostheses is covered by Berger and Cooney III elsewhere in this issue.

Soft tissue rebalancing

At the conclusion of the previous procedures, meticulous soft tissue reconstruction [43] and ECU rebalancing is paramount to the success of any operation involving RA of the DRUJ [13]. The remaining DRUJ capsule is usually inadequate for repair. The ulnar limb of the extensor retinaculum therefore is used for dorsal capsular reconstruction and is sutured over the distal ulna palmar to the reduced ECU tendon. Several investigators advocate using the extensor retinaculum to reduce and stabilize the ECU tendon [3,4,24,41,52]. In the authors' method, the proximal half of the radial aspect of the extensor retinaculum may be used as a sling around the ECU tendon and sutured to the more distal portion of the retinaculum rather than to itself. This creates a loose sling rather than a noose [24,52] (see Fig. 6), and the distal half may be repaired back dorsal to the extensor tendons to prevent bowstringing. Indications for ECRL to ECU transfer are in patients who have MCP ulnar drift with a passively correctable wrist radial deviation deformity and spared radiocarpal joint [24]. It is also useful in patients who lack the ability or can only weakly actively ulnar deviate the wrist. The ECRL to ECU transfer may be performed by dividing the ECRL at the base of the second metacarpal bone and routing it dorsal to the extensor tendons and suturing it to the repositioned ECU tendon [3,20].

If after the DRUJ procedure is performed there is still decreased forearm rotation, the problem may lie in the PRUJ of the elbow. This may have to be addressed [2] with possible debridement or radial head resection [17].

Summary

The DRUJ frequently is involved in RA and can be a source of major disability. Nonoperative treatment consists of adequate hand/occupational therapy, judicious splinting, and pharmacologic management. If unacceptable pain and dysfunction persists or if there is tendon rupture, surgery is indicated. Surgical treatment ranges from debridement and soft tissue balancing if the joint is preserved to osseous procedures ranging from Darrach resection, Sauve-Kapandji procedure, hemiresection, to distal ulna replacement. Tendon ruptures usually require tendon transfers.

If an osseous procedure is required, the authors prefer the Sauve-Kapandji procedure in the younger, active adult. Darrach distal ulna resection is recommended for the older, sedentary patient. For either procedure, if there is evidence of pre-existing radiocarpal instability, partial or total wrist arthrodesis or arthroplasty should be a concomitant procedure.

References

[1] Clawson MC, Stern PJ. The distal radioulnar joint complex in rheumatoid arthritis: an overview. Hand Clin 1991;7(2):373–81.

[2] O'Donovan TM, Ruby LK. The distal radioulnar joint in rheumatoid arthritis. Hand Clin 1989;5(2): 249–56.

[3] Ryu J, Patel SM. Rheumatoid arthritis-soft tissue reconstruction. In: Trumble TE, editor. Hand surgery update 3. Rosemont (IL): American Society for Surgery of the Hand; 2003. p. 535–51.

[4] Feldon P, Terrono AL, Nalebuff EA, et al. Rheumatoid arthritis and other connective tissue diseases. In: Green DP, Hotchkiss RN, Pederson WC, et al, editors. Green's operative hand surgery. 5th edition. Philadelphia: Elsevier Churchill Livingstone; 2005. p. 2049–136.

[5] Goldfarb CA, Stern PJ. Rheumatoid arthritis-skeletal reconstruction. In: Trumble TE, editor. Hand surgery update 3. Rosemont (IL): American Society for Surgery of the Hand; 2002. p. 525–33.

[6] Leak RS, Rayan GM, Arthur RE. Longitudinal radiographic analysis of rheumatoid arthritis in the hand and wrist. J Hand Surg 2003;28A:427–34.

[7] Stuart PR, Berger RA. The dorsopalmar stability of the distal radioulnar joint. J Hand Surg 2000;25A: 689–99.

[8] Adams BD. Distal radioulnar joint. In: Trumble TE, editor. Hand surgery update 3. Rosemont: American Society for Surgery of the Hand; 2003. p. 147–57.

[9] Palmer AK, Werner FW. The triangular fibrocartilage complex of the wrist—anatomy and function. J Hand Surg 1981;6A:153–62.

[10] Drobner WS, Hausman MR. The distal radioulnar joint. Hand Clin 1992;8:631–44.

[11] Weiler PJ, Bogoch ER. Kinematics of the distal radioulnar joint in rheumatoid arthritis: an in vivo study using centrode analysis. J Hand Surg 1995; 20A:937–43.

[12] Cracchiolo A 3rd, Marmor L. Resection of the distal ulna in rheumatoid arthritis. Arthritis Rheum 1969; 12(4):415–22.

[13] Backdahl M. The caput ulnae syndrome in rheumatoid arthritis. A study of the morphology, abnormal anatomy and clinical picture. Acta Rheumatol Scand 1963;(Suppl 5):1–75.

[14] Spinner M, Kaplan EB. Extensor carpi ulnaris: its relationship to the stability of the distal radio-ulnar joint. Clin Orthop 1970;68:124–9.

[15] Vaughan-Jackson OJ. Attritional rupture of tendons in the rheumatoid hand. J Bone Joint Surg 1958;40A:1431.

[16] Vaughan-Jackson OJ. Rupture of tendons by attrition at the inferior radioulnar joint. Report of two cases. J Bone Joint Surg 1948;30B:528.

[17] Clayton ML. Surgical treatment at the wrist in rheumatoid arthritis. J Bone Joint Surg 1965;47A: 741–50.

[18] Millender LH, Nalebuff EA, Albin R, et al. Dorsal tenosynovectomy and tendon transfer in the rheumatoid hand. J Bone Joint Surg 1974;56A:601–10.

[19] Moore JR, Weiland AJ, Valdata L. Tendon ruptures in the rheumatoid hand: analysis of treatment and functional results in 60 patients. J Hand Surg 1987; 12A:9–14.

[20] Thirupathi RG, Ferlic DC, Clayton ML. Dorsal wrist synovectomy in rheumatoid arthritis—a long-term study. J Hand Surg 1983;8A:848–56.

[21] Berger RA. Instructional course lecture 227. Injuries of the distal radioulnar joint. American Academy of

Orthopaedic Surgeons 72nd Annual Meeting, February 24, 2005, Washington, DC.

[22] Freiberg RA, Weinstein A. The scallop sign and spontaneous rupture of finger extensor tendons in rheumatoid arthritics. Clin Orthop 1972;83: 128–30.

[23] Alderman AK, Ubel PA, Kim HM, et al. Surgical management of the rheumatoid hand: consensus and controversy among rheumatologists and hand surgeons. J Rheumatol 2003;30(7):1464–72.

[24] Blank JE, Cassidy C. The distal radioulnar joint in rheumatoid arthritis. Hand Clin 1996;12(3): 499–513.

[25] Mandl LA, Galvin DH, Bosch JP, et al. Metacarpophalangeal arthroplasty in rheumatoid arthritis: what determines satisfaction with surgery? J Rheumatol 2002;29:2488–91.

[26] Buck-Gramcko D. Denervation of the wrist joint. J Hand Surg 1977;2A:54–61.

[27] Brumfield R Jr, Kuschner SH, Gellman H, et al. Results of dorsal wrist synovectomies in the rheumatoid hand. J Hand Surg 1990;15A:733–5.

[28] Mannerfelt LG. Tendon transfers in surgery of the rheumatoid hand. Hand Clin 1988;4:309–16.

[29] Rana NA, Taylor AR. Excision of distal end of the ulna in rheumatoid arthritis. J Bone Joint Surg 1973;55B:96–105.

[30] Melone CP Jr, Taras JS. Distal ulna resection, extensor carpi ulnaris tenodesis, and dorsal synovectomy for the rheumatoid wrist. Hand Clin 1991;7(2): 335–43.

[31] Nalebuff EA, Patel MR. Flexor digitorum sublimis transfer for multiple extensor tendon ruptures in rheumatoid arthritis. Plast Reconstr Surg 1973;52: 530–3.

[32] Darrach W. Anterior dislocation of the ulna. Ann Surg 1912;56:802–3.

[33] Darrach W. Fractures of the lower extremity of the radius: diagnosis and treatment. JAMA 1927;89: 1683–5.

[34] Dingman PV. Resection of the distal end of the ulna (Darrach operation); an end result study of twenty four cases. J Bone Joint Surg 1952;34A:893–900.

[35] Bowers WH. Distal radioulnar joint arthroplasty: the hemiresection-interposition technique. J Hand Surg 1985;10A:169–78.

[36] Watson HK, Ryu JY, Burgess RC. Matched distal ulnar resection. J Hand Surg 1986;11A:812–7.

[37] Sauve Kapandji. Nouvelle technique de traitement chirurgical des luxations recidivantes isolees de l'extremite inferieure du cubitas. J Chir (Paris) 1936;47:589–94.

[38] Cooney WP IV. Instructional course lecture 227. Injuries of the distal radioulnar joint. American Academy of Orthopaedic Surgeons 72nd Annual Meeting, February 24, 2005, Washington, DC.

[39] Liebolt FL. A new procedure for the treatment of luxation of distal end of the ulna. J Bone Joint Surg 1953;35A:261–2.

[40] Smith-Peterson MN, Aufranc OE, Larson CB. Useful surgical procedures for rheumatoid arthritis involving joints of the upper extremity. Arch Surg 1943;46:764–70.

[41] Posner MA, Ambrose L. Excision of the distal ulna in rheumatoid arthritis. Hand Clin 1991;7(2): 383–90.

[42] Leslie BM, Carlson G, Ruby LK. Results of extensor carpi ulnaris tenodesis in the rheumatoid wrist undergoing a distal ulnar excision. J Hand Surg 1990;15A:547–51.

[43] Newmeyer WL, Green DP. Rupture of digital extensor tendons following distal ulnar resection. J Bone Joint Surg 1982;64A:178–82.

[44] Fraser KE, Diao E, Peimer CA, et al. Comparative results of resection of the distal ulna in rheumatoid arthritis and post-traumatic conditions. J Hand Surg 1999;24B:667–70.

[45] Van Gemert AM, Spauwen PH. Radiological evaluation of the long-term effects of resection of the distal ulna in rheumatoid arthritis. J Hand Surg 1994; 19B:330–3.

[46] Black RM, Boswick JA Jr, Wiedel J. Dislocation of the wrist in rheumatoid arthritis. The relationship to distal ulna resection. Clin Orthop 1977;124:184–8.

[47] Gainor BJ, Schaberg J. The rheumatoid wrist after resection of the distal ulna. J Hand Surg 1985;10A: 837–44.

[48] Pirela-Cruz MA, Firoozbakhsh K, Moneim MS. Ulnar translation of the carpus in rheumatoid arthritis: an analysis of five determination methods. J Hand Surg 1993;18A:299–306.

[49] DiBenedetto MR, Lubbers LM, Coleman CR. Long-term results of the minimal resection Darrach procedure. J Hand Surg 1991;16A:445–50.

[50] Goncalves D. Correction of disorders of the distal radio-ulnar joint by artificial pseudarthrosis of the ulna. J Bone Joint Surg 1974;56B:462–4.

[51] Chamay A, Della Santa D, Vilaseca A. Radiolunate arthrodesis. Factor of stability for the rheumatoid wrist. Ann Chir Main 1983;2(1):5–17.

[52] Adams BD. Distal radioulnar joint instability. In: Green DP, Hotchkiss RN, Pederson WC, et al, editors. Green's operative hand surgery. 5th edition. Philadelphia: Elsevier Churchill Livingstone; 2005. p. 605–44.

[53] Bieber EJ, Linscheid RL, Dobyns JH, et al. Failed distal ulna resections. J Hand Surg 1998;13A: 193–200.

[54] Tulipan DJ, Eaton RG, Eberhart RE. The Darrach procedure defended: technique redefined and long-term follow-up. J Hand Surg 1991;16A:438–44.

[55] Rowland SA. Stabilization of the ulnar side of the rheumatoid wrist, following radiocarpal Swanson's implant arthroplasty and resection of the distal ulna. Bull Hosp Joint Dis Orthop Inst 1984;44: 442–8.

[56] Tsai TM, Stilwell JH. Repair of chronic subluxation of the distal radioulnar joint (ulnar dorsal) using

flexor carpi ulnaris tendon. J Hand Surg 1984;9B: 289–94.

[57] Breen TF, Jupiter JB. Extensor carpi ulnaris and flexor carpi ulnaris tenodesis of the unstable distal ulna. J Hand Surg 1989;14A:612–7.

[58] Carter PB, Stuart PR. The Sauve-Kapandji procedure for post-traumatic disorders of the distal radio-ulnar joint. J Bone Joint Surg 2000;82B:1013–8.

[59] Kleinman WB, Greenberg JA. Salvage of the failed Darrach procedure. J Hand Surg 1995;20A:951–8.

[60] Wolfe SW, Mih AD, Hotchkiss RN, et al. Wide excision of the distal ulna: a multicenter case study. J Hand Surg 1998;23A:222–8.

[61] Steindler A. Orthopaedic operations. Springfield (IL): Charles C. Thomas; 1940. p. 492.

[62] Vincent KA, Szabo RM, Agee JM. The Sauve-Kapandji procedure for reconstruction of the rheumatoid distal radioulnar joint. J Hand Surg 1993; 18A:978–83.

[63] Fujita S, Masada K, Takeuchi E, et al. Modified Sauve-Kapandji procedure for disorders of the distal radioulnar joint in patients with rheumatoid arthritis. J Bone Joint Surg 2005;87A:134–9.

[64] Adams BD. Instructional course lecture 227. Injuries of the distal radioulnar joint. American Academy of Orthopaedic Surgeons 72nd Annual Meeting, February 24, 2005, Washington, DC.

[65] Rothwell AG, O'Neill L, Cragg K. Sauve-Kapandji procedure for disorders of the distal radioulnar joint: a simplified technique. J Hand Surg 1996;21A: 771–7.

[66] Millroy P, Coleman S, Ivers R. The Sauve-Kapandji operation. J Hand Surg 1992;17B:411–4.

[67] Minami A, Kato H, Iwasaki N. Modification of the Sauve-Kapandji procedure with extensor carpi ulnaris tenodesis. J Hand Surg 2000;25A: 1080–4.

[68] Lamey DM, Fernandez DL. Results of the modified Sauve-Kapandji procedure in the treatment of chronic posttraumatic derangement of the distal radioulnar joint. J Bone Joint Surg 1998;80A: 1758–69.

[69] Taleisnik J. The Sauve-Kapandji procedure. Clin Orthop 1992;275:110–23.

[70] Lichtman DM, Ganocy TK, Kim DC. The indications for and techniques and outcomes of ablative procedures of the distal ulna: the Darrach resection, hemiresection, matched resection and Sauve-Kapandji procedure. Hand Clin 1988;14: 265–77.

[71] Sanders RA, Frederick HA, Hontas RB. The Sauve-Kapandji procedure: a salvage operation for the distal radioulnar joint. J Hand Surg 1991; 16A:1125–9.

ELSEVIER
SAUNDERS

Hand Clin 21 (2005) 591–601

HAND
CLINICS

Hemiresection Arthroplasty of the Distal Radioulnar Joint

Keith A. Glowacki, MD[a,b],*

[a]Advanced Orthopaedic Centers, 7650 East Parham Road, Richmond, VA 23294, USA
[b]Virginia Commonwealth University, Medical College of Virginia, 1200 East Broad Street,
Richmond, VA 23298-0153, USA

Painful disorders of the distal radioulnar joint (DRUJ) and the triangular fibrocartilage complex (TFCC) are becoming recognized and treated more frequently. A systemic approach to these often difficult to diagnose problems can lead to the appropriate treatment, and if necessary, the appropriate surgical intervention. This issue devotes its attention to wrist arthritis; therefore, the focus of this article is on arthritis of the DRUJ treated specifically by hemiresection arthroplasty of the DRUJ. Arthroplasty techniques, in general, of the DRUJ are grouped into several categories. There are excisional arthroplasties, complete and partial, which include the Darrach procedure, the Feldon wafer procedure, the matched (Watson) resection, and the hemiresection interposition (Bower) arthroplasty [1–5]. Also included are ulnar shortening and replacement arthroplasty. There are now sufficient studies on most of these techniques to give excellent comparison and functional outcomes [6–21]. This allows the surgeon to make the appropriate choice of procedure, based on a thorough knowledge of the patient and their functional demands.

Anatomy

The anatomy of the DRUJ and its supporting ligaments is complex. During the last few years important kinematic studies on the normal wrist have increased understanding considerably [22,23].

A thorough knowledge of the anatomy is necessary to manage the pathologic conditions that arise. Stability is achieved through articular contact and ligamentous stabilizers. The DRUJ articulation is a trochoid one, similar to that of the proximal radioulnar joint. The shallow sigmoid articular notch has dimensions 1.5 cm dorsal to volar and 1 cm proximal to distal. The notch has three distinct margins (dorsal, distal, and palmar). The dorsal margin is acutely angular in cross-section and the palmar less so. The carpal distal margin is the junction between the notch and the distally facing lunate facet. The two are separated by the attachment of the triangular fibrocartilage to the radius. The articulation of the ulnar head with the sigmoid notch is not congruous in as much as the radius (Fig. 1) [24]. The shallow arc of the sigmoid notch is greater than that of the ulnar convexity. Because of the different radii of curvature there is a sliding/rolling component with forearm pronation and supination. In the normal ligamentous support the two surfaces allow a dorsal volar translation. This translation has been measured as 2.8 mm dorsal and 5.4 mm palmar in 0° rotation position. During this midrange the sigmoid notch accepts 60°–80° of the 130° articular convexity. In the extremes of rotation, however, less than 10% of the surface may be in contact with the dorsal or palmar margin of the notch. Because of the less constrained articular surface, the ligamentous stabilizers play a much more important role in this joint. The TFCC (as described by Palmar) [25–28] contains the annular ligaments, the articular disc, a meniscus homolog, and the ulnar collateral ligaments. The ulnar collateral ligaments suspend the lunate and triquetral carpal bones to the ulna (ulnolunate and ulnotriquetral).

---

* Advanced Orthopaedic Centers, 7650 East Parham Road, Richmond, VA 23294, USA.
E-mail address: kglowacki@aocortho.com

doi:10.1016/j.hcl.2005.08.002

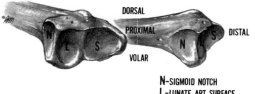

N-SIGMOID NOTCH
L-LUNATE ART. SURFACE
S-SCAPHOID ART. SURFACE

Fig. 1. The bony anatomy of the distal radius and the distal radioulnar joint. (*From* Green's operative hand surgery, volume 1, 4th edition. New York: Elsevier; 1998; with permission.)

The TFCC attaches the radius to the ulna and is part of an extensive fibrous system that arises from the carpal margin of the sigmoid notch, cups the lunate and triquetral bones, and reaches the volar base of the fifth metacarpal (Fig. 2) [29].

Stability of the radioulnar and carpal unit is influenced additionally by the configuration of the sigmoid notch, the slope of the ulnar dome, the interosseous membrane, the extensor retinaculum, the dynamic forces of the extensor carpi ulnaris (ECU), pronator quadratus, and the dorsal carpal ligamentous complex. The triangular fibrocartilage complex provides a continuous gliding surface across the entire distal two forearm bones for carpal flexion, extension, and translational movements. It also provides a flexible mechanism for stable rotational movements of the radius around the ulnar axis. It suspends the ulnar carpus from the dorsal ulnar base of the radius, and it cushions forces transmitted through the ulnar carpal axis. The peripheral margins of the triangular fibrocartilage consist of thick lamellar collagen adapted to bare tensile loading, often referred to as the dorsal and palmar radioulnar ligament. It also solidly connects the ulnar axis to the volar carpus. The portion of the TFCC called the triangular fibrocartilage is 1–2 mm thick at its base and is attached to the distal margin of the sigmoid notch. Viewed from within the radioulnar joint, the styloid attachment seems folded. The intra-articular fold and its vascular hilum have been termed the ligamentum subcruetum. The triangular fibrocartilage has a thin central portion occasionally referred to as the articular disc. It is chondroid-type fibrocartilage and the type of tissue that bears compressive loads. The distribution of forces is important in understanding abnormalities of the DRUJ. Compressive force across the carpal ulnar articulation is partially transmitted through the center of the TFCC to the ulnar

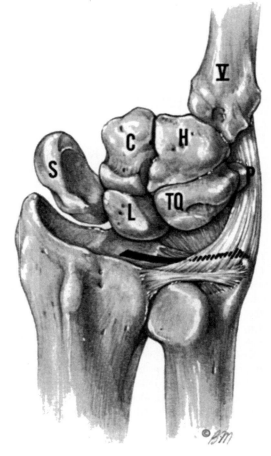

Fig. 2. The ulnar collateral ligaments, including the ulnolunate and ulnotriquetral ligaments. The meniscal Homologue, the radioulnar ligaments, and the TFCC are shown cupping the ulnocarpal bones in this anatomic picture. (*From* Green's operative hand surgery, volume 1, 4th edition. New York: Elsevier; 1998; with permission.)

dome. This force tends to have a separating effect on the radius and ulna. The TFCC converts some of this compressive force into a tensile force with its lamellar peripheral collagen arrangement [30,31]. The pronator quadratus muscle action and the interosseous membrane help with this functional demand. The rest of the load is taken by the ulnar dome. Palmar and Warner have shown experimentally that in a neutral variant 80% of the static axial load is borne by the radius, whereas 20% is borne by the ulna. If the ulnar length is increased 2.5 mm the load borne by the ulnar dome increases 40% [26].

Mechanics

The rotational movement of the radius–TFCC complex over the ulnar dome allows various loading scenarios. This variable loading may account for the location and nature of tears seen in the TFCC by Chidgey [32] and others [26,33]. The marginal ligaments of the TFCC are important, not only in load transference from the carpus to the ulna but also in the stability of the radioulnar joint. In extremes of rotation the compressive forces between the radius and ulna are resisted by the reciprocal tensile forces developed within the TFCC marginal ligaments. Numerous studies now support how this complex functions [32–35]. The two structures (TFCC and ulnocarpal ligaments) are morphologically distinct and have individual roles, even though the complex functions as a unit. The role of the ulnocarpal ligaments is to provide a stable connection between the ulna and the volar ulnar carpus. This ligament resists dorsal displacement of the distal ulna relative to the carpus. Destruction of this ligament, as is seen commonly by attenuation in rheumatoid arthritis, allows volar displacement of the carpus in relation to the distal ulna, a condition that is even more obvious in pronation. Disruption of any of these elements, the TFCC, the radioulnar ligaments, the ulnocarpal ligaments, the pronator quadratus, the ECU subsheath, and the interosseous membrane, may lead to arthrosis, limited motion, or instability.

Indications

There are several procedures that may be grouped under the heading arthroplasty of the DRUJ. A subgroup of these procedures is known as partial resection arthroplasties or hemi-arthroplasties. This article focuses on the partial resection arthroplasty known as the Bower hemiresection arthroplasty [2]. Partial resection arthroplasty may be viewed as an attempt to address selectively the pathology yet retain elements of the articulation important to its function. There is an element of retaining structure of the ulnar column and its ligamentous attachments to the radius and carpus in this procedure. The ulnar shaft styloid axis is kept intact. Hemiresection arthroplasty is indicated primarily in the treatment of posttraumatic, degenerative, and rheumatoid arthritis of the DRUJ. Although these types of arthritis are etiologically different, they present similar treatment problems conservative and surgical.

The differential diagnosis for pain at the DRUJ includes arthritic deformities, instability, ulnocarpal impaction, acute subluxation, chronic subluxation or dislocations, chronic instability of the DRUJ, and inflammatory conditions (ie, rheumatoid arthritis).

Examination

Arthritis of the DRUJ causes significant disability and severe pain. The physician must correlate the history, physical examination, and diagnostic data to be able to make a well defined clinical decision on how best to treat the patient and improve their quality of life. Arthritis of the DRUJ primarily presents with pain. There is crepitation with pronation and supination. The history would be a gradual onset with increasing frequency over many years.

Included in this decision are the demands of the patient, their work history, their age, and their hand dominance. The physical examination should include the age, dominance, characteristics of the symptoms, range of motion, pronation and supination, flexion and extension, and comparison to the contralateral side. Crepitation on the piano key maneuver and testing the patient's distal DRUJ with the elbow flexed at a 90° angle in 3° of motion, full pronation and supination, and neutral is necessary. Palpation along the areas of the triangular fibrocartilage, the foveal region, and the ulnar styloid are all performed. Other tests include the lunotriquetral sheer and shuck test and an impaction test in maximal wrist extension with force across the palm. All can reveal provocative findings of pain. Palpation of the ECU tendon sheath is done, as is resisted pronation to elicit any tendon subluxation. Diagnostic injection of an anesthetic or steroid also is used in assessing which area is contributing to the patient's source of pain and disability. Pre- and postinjection improvement of grip strength and pain in the possible area of the patient's pathology is favorable. Fluoroscopy can be used to guide the needle to the area of pain. This allows for more reproducible results and diagnosis. The patient frequently is asked to duplicate the motion that causes their symptoms.

Diagnostic studies

Standardized radiographs are extremely important in the DRUJ. Assessing ulnar positive and negative variance becomes important in stylocarpal impingement and in ulnocarpal impaction syndrome. A standard zero rotation PA and lateral radiograph in neutral are obtained. Motion series can be added, including ulnar deviation and radial deviation. A clenched fist can be added to supplement these initial radiographs. Findings include narrowing of the joint space in the DRUJ, sclerosis of the articular surfaces, and spur and cyst formation. MRI, including an arthrogram to supplement, is used specifically for ligamentous injury, such as the lunotriquetral, TFCC, and scapholunate ligaments. With increasing age, arthritis is found more commonly. This also correlates with increasing findings of ligament tears, and the true pathology sometimes can be somewhat questionable. Several studies have shown up to 50% of individuals over the age of 60 years may have TFCC tears that are asymptomatic [27,36]. Computed tomography with 3-D reconstruction has proven useful in evaluating subluxation of the distal radioulnar with axial cuts in pronation and supination. It also can evaluate thoroughly the surfaces of the DRUJ that may be arthritic. The ability to manipulate these images, computed tomography, and MR may become used more frequently in an educational role to the patient in an office setting and in simulating surgical procedures. Other diagnostic techniques include arthroscopy to supplement the findings of MRI and arthrography. Because arthritic conditions frequently are accompanied by associated ligamentous tears, arthroscopy can be used to assess the quality of cartilage before performing a hemiresection. The relevance of positive arthrograms has been questioned because of a high incidence of symmetric lesions. There is also a poor correlation with physical examination in some arthrographic findings. Injection of a contrast material in a triple versus single injection

arthrography is debated. Because this is performed most commonly by radiologists without the presence of a surgeon, the benefit of having a direct view of the arthrogram is lost. Some surgeons perform their own arthrogram for this reason.

MRI increasingly uses enhancing materials to increase visualization of soft-tissue and bony pathology. Use of extremity coils and stronger magnets are creating much better and clearer images of the wrist ligaments with MRI.

Arthroscopy increasingly is being used in the wrist and other small joints in the hand over the last 5–10 years. The direct visualization of these injuries has no equivalent in determining pathology. It also can be diagnostic and therapeutic. In this present age of patient care, however, frequently it would be difficult without an MRI or other diagnostic tests to do a simple arthroscopy as a pure diagnostic tool. Arthritic disorders are still somewhat limited in their treatment with arthroscopy. Recent articles have revealed benefit by doing a Feldon wafer resection arthroscopically with TFCC debridement [21]. The DRUJ is a less predictably entered joint. It is extremely small and difficult to insert the arthroscope. As the tools and the applications increase, someday this may be more common.

Surgical approach

The keys to exposure are the ECU tendon and the extensor digiti minimi (EDM) tendons. As the ECU tendon enters the retinacular compartment, it lies directly on top of the ulnar styloid in any position of forearm rotation. The EDM changes from the muscle to tendon as it enters this retinacular compartment. This tendon lies along the radial attachment of the TFCC. For exposure of the major portion of the ulnar articular surface the

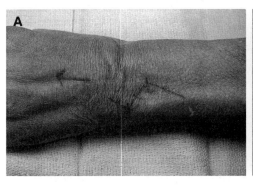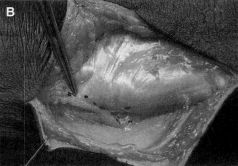

Fig. 3. (*A*) The dorsal approach. The arrow points to the patient's hand. (*B*) The ulnar nerve with the forceps and the dotted marks on the ulnar aspect. There is an additional ulnar nerve in the soft tissues in the bottom right corner.

procedure is begun with the wrist in full pronation. The incision begins laterally three fingerbreadths proximal to the styloid along the ulnar shaft and gently curves around the distal side of the head to end dorsally at the mid-carpus. Further extension can be performed distally, as this incision can be curved back ulnarly (Fig. 3A,B). The incision lies just dorsal to the dorsal branches of the ulnar sensory nerve, which must be found and protected with retraction or vessel loops during the procedure. Dorsal veins also are retracted, and the dissection is carried to the obliquely lying extensor retinacular fibers. Beneath the proximal border of the retinaculum the capsule of the ulnar head passes between the EDM and the ECU or fifth and sixth compartments.

The proximal and ulnar half of the extensor retinaculum is reflexed radially to uncover the ECU and EDM tendons. The base of this flap is the septum between the EDM and extensor digitorum comminus (EDC) compartment. Care is taken to maintain the EDC compartment intact.

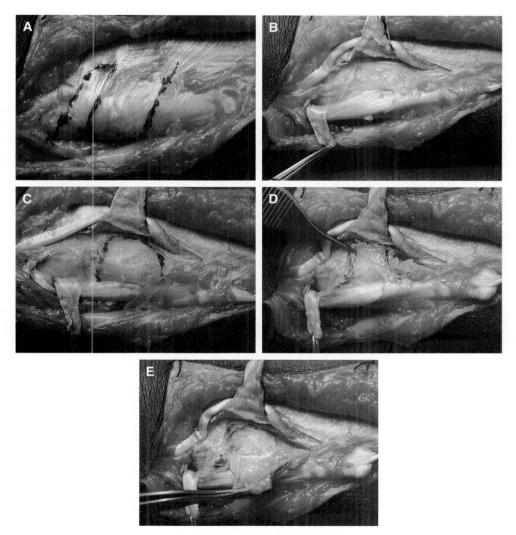

Fig. 4. (*A*) The proximal radial-based and the distal ulnar-based retinacular flaps that potentially are to be used to sling the ECU and to cover the capsule. (*B*) Those flaps opened, taking careful attention not to violate most of the ECU sheath. (*C*) The capsular incision marked. (*D*) That capsular incision made. (*E*) On opening that capsular incision, the ulnar head is exposed.

The EDM is retracted to reveal the dorsal margin of the sigmoid notch of the radius and the TFCC. The capsule then is sharply detached from the radius with a 1-mm cuff for later repair (Fig. 4A–E). As the capsule then is reflected toward the ulna, the ulnar head is exposed. A small lamina spreader or retractor can be placed to view the sigmoid notch. To better expose the underside of the TFCC, the forearm could be brought into neutral rotation and a small retractor placed, pulling the capsule distally. Further exposing the TFCC, as this is commonly debrided during the case of any central tearing, is done by releasing the EDM and ECU from the retinacular compartment. This can be done by reflecting the distal half of the extensor retinaculum opposite that of the first flap in an ulnar direction with an ulnar-based flap. The retinaculum is divided along the EDM septum, and the base of this flap is the attachment of the ECU compartment nearest the ulna. The ECU should be released fully only if its pathology is involved; otherwise, it should be kept unviolated in its sixth compartment and subperiosteally dissected from the ulnar shaft. This is critical because of its stabilizing function.

When the EDM and the ECU are reflected to either side one observes the transverse fibers of the dorsal radiotriquetral ligament. This ligament may be incised along its course parallel to the fibers to look at the lunate and triquetral surfaces within the radiocarpal joint. A triangular-based flap may be elevated. For exposure of the styloid the forearm is carried into full supination with the groove of the ECU used to mark its dorsal base. The reflected capsule may be used as an interpositional flap on performing a partial distal ulna resection. The ECU should be returned to its groove, and the first retinacular flap can be used as a stabilizing sling for the tendon if necessary (Fig. 5).

The intact DRUJ surfaces and the ulnocarpal joint structures cannot be explored fully by a single approach because of the close contact of the radius and the ulna. This approach allows visualization of 60% of the ulnar head, carpal base of the TFCC, lunotriquetral ligament, triquetrum, prestyloid recess, and most of the DRUJ synovial cavity. If carefully dissected and replaced, none of this exposure should alter the mechanics or stability. It is the resection of the distal ulna that uncouples the rotational unit of the DRUJ. This leads to the instability problems and impingement frequently seen as a complication of this procedure.

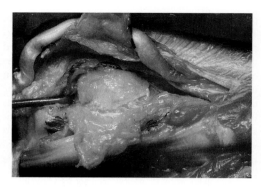

Fig. 5. The subperiosteally elevated portion of the ECU off of the distal ulna so as to prepare for the osteotomy. The freer is in the radiocarpal joint proximal to the TFCC.

Hemiresection

In performing a hemiresection arthroplasty there is no need to enter the radiocarpal joint or expose the carpal surface of the TFCC unless a pathologic tear is suspected. The retinacular flaps that were developed can be used for augmentation of the deficient TFCC if necessary (the distal flap) or in stabilization of the ECU tendon (the proximal flap). If at all possible, the ECU sheath should not be removed from its retinacular compartment if it is stable. Only in cases in which instability occurs should this be stabilized with a flap. Subperiosteally reflecting off of the ulna allows for visualization of the ulnar head and distal ulnar head.

The DRUJ capsule then is divided, exposing the articular surface, at which time a synovectomy may be performed. The ulnar articular surface and the subchondral bone then are removed with a combination of an oscillating saw, osteotome, or rongeurs. The most common pitfall in this area is to inadequately remove the distal ulnar articular surface. One needs to make sure that with pronation and supination they get the entire articular surface, the osteophytes around the sigmoid notch, and the ulnar head articular surfaces. The most difficult portion to remove is the volar portion of the head. The TFCC can be visualized on removing the head, and at this point most central TFCC tears can be debrided if necessary (Fig. 6A,B).

At this point one can assess the possibility of ulna stylocarpal impingement. Usually this is assessed preoperatively with appropriate radiographs also. On compressing the radial and ulnar

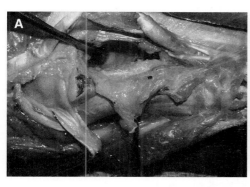
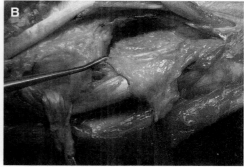

Fig. 6. (*A*) The early portion shows the most dorsal radial aspect of the distal ulna removed. (*B*) On rotating the ulna through a full pronation and supination, the full hemiresection is achieved. In the depths of the wound the freer points to distal radius aspect of the DRUJ.

shafts with the wrist ulnarly deviated, if there is any question about the ulnar styloid impinging on the carpal bones, the ulna then should be shortened. The shortening can be done through the metaphyseal base at the site of the ulnar head or more proximally with plate application. The usual fixation is with several 2.0 or 3.0 nonabsorbable sutures (Fig. 7) [37]. The next step is to place in the resected ulnar space material, usually tendon, as an interposed bulky material to maintain radial ulnar shaft separation. This also is meant to prohibit impingement in cases in which the ulna is a zero variant (palmaris longus or ECU/FCU tendon strip) (Fig. 8A–C).

The ECU compartment then is replaced into the area. Sometimes a portion of the distal retinacular flap is sewn down into the capsule to maintain the interpositional material. If the ECU compartment needs to be stabilized it is then performed (Fig. 9A–D). If no shortening is performed, a postoperative short arm bulky dressing with dorsal and palmar plaster splints is applied. Finger motion is encouraged within 3–5 days with early anti-edema and therapy. At 2 weeks the sutures are removed and the patient is placed into a short arm cast or wrist splint for 2–4 more weeks.

If an ulnar shortening is performed with the hemiresection, the initial immobilization is a long arm sugar tong or long arm splint controlling forearm rotation. This then is converted to a short arm cast with interosseous molding at 2–4 weeks. This allows slightly more rotation but it is important that the short arm cast have good interosseous molding. A wrist splint then is used from 6 weeks to full use over the next 4 weeks. The patient is assessed at every visit for

osteosynthesis with radiographs and at that point may remove any protective splinting. This typically takes 10–12 weeks.

The surgical alternatives for conditions of post-traumatic, degenerative, and inflammatory arthritis of the DRUJ are excision of the distal end of the ulna, known as the Darrach procedure

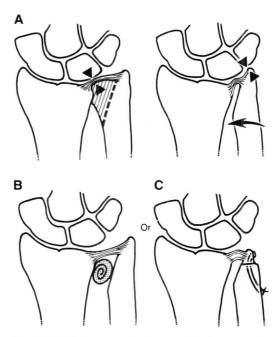

Fig. 7. (*A–C*) In cases of stylocarpal impingement the ulna is shortened, either (as this shows) through an interosseous wiring technique or as can be performed with two anchors through drill holes of a nonabsorbable suture. (*From* Green's operative hand surgery, volume 1, 4th edition. New York: Elsevier; 1998; with permission.)

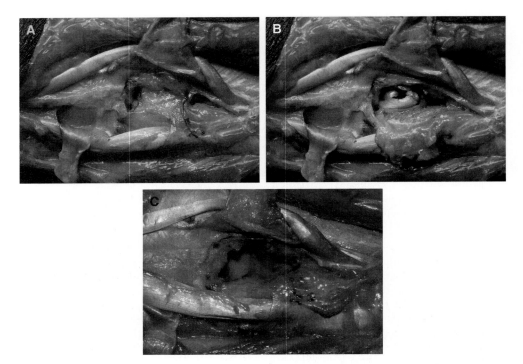

Fig. 8. (*A*) The previous DRUJ capsular flap (see Fig. 4*C*). This flap is shown sewn down to the volar capsule and tissue after the resection covering the hemiresection. (*B*) The palmaris longus tendon sewn typically to a previously placed stitch along the volar capsule to secure it, followed by closure of the capsule over top in (*C*).

with one of the many modifications of this technique to stabilize the ulnar stump, the hemiresection arthroplasty, the Sauve-Kapandji procedure, and other salvage-type procedures, including a one-bone forearm and a more proximal distal ulnar resection. Replacement arthroplasty increasingly is used also. This article primarily focuses on the hemiresection arthroplasty technique, its most appropriate indication, pitfalls, and salvage techniques used in the event of failure of treatment.

The problems associated with the Darrach operation were improved on by Bowers in 1985 [2] and Watson [3]. Both of these procedures proposed a similar philosophy and a technique in a partial resection of the distal ulna. The ulnar styloid axis and the soft-tissue attachment to the TFCC were left intact. These were operations designed to handle the shaft instability that was found after many Darrach procedures. More attention to detail was required with these procedures. Adequate resection is imperative to prevent postoperative impingement between the remaining ulnar shaft and the radius. This is the most common source of continued pain and

failure of the procedure. Despite these techniques, radioulnar convergence still occurs. These initial studies were performed primarily in patients who had rheumatoid arthritis. Bowers reported on 38 cases, and 27 of 38 were rheumatoid [2]. Watson reported on 48 cases, 34 of which were rheumatoid [3]. Other studies [14–16,18,38–40] have added experience in combined series revealing primarily patients who have rheumatoid arthritis at 42%, patients who have instability at 29%, ulnocarpal impingement 21%, primary osteoarthritis 5%, and 3% other traumatic problems. In this multi-series review 76% of the patients were pain free and 24% had mild pain. Two percent of these patients were treated with repeat operation for stylocarpal impingement [6].

The purpose of this procedure is to obtain relief of pain by complete resection of only the articular prominence, leaving the ulnar column intact. This procedure was an outgrowth of what Dingman described as the best of the Darrach procedures, in which there was minimal resection followed by some regeneration of the ulnar shaft within the retained sleeve of the periosteum. An interposition of tendon, muscle, or capsule is

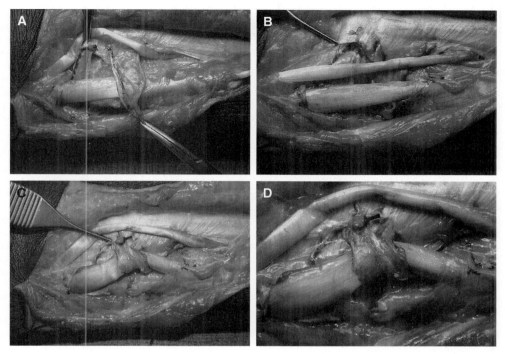

Fig. 9. (*A*) With no need to stabilize the ECU, the previous ulnar and the previous proximal and distal retinacular flaps can be sewn back, leaving the fifth compartment transposed. (*B*) Those retinaculum sewn in place. Note the proximal stability of the ECU tendon on the right side. (*C, D*) A sling and close-up using the proximal radial-based retinaculum. This sling is slightly tighter than standard, but in the case of a rheumatoid, this would be used for stabilization.

placed in the vacant DRUJ synovial cavity to limit contact of the radial and ulnar shafts in convergence. The procedure supposes an intact or reconstructible TFCC. It should not be used in situations in which ulnar variance is positive unless the ulna is shortened as part of the procedure. This avoids the common problem of stylocarpal impingement. Most cases in patients who have rheumatoid arthritis with TFCC have unreconstructable TFCCs. Here a modified Darrach procedure coupled with radiolunate arthrodesis is a good choice; another alternative is a Sauve-Kapandji procedure. An additional contraindication is preoperative evidence of ulnocarpal translation. The operation has one inherent problem. If the articular surfaces are removed sufficiently, they unload the ulnocarpal articulation, changing the normal force distribution in the wrist. The normal articular dome provides a stable seat for the radius to ride in its rotational arc, and its absence allows the two shafts to come together. If on a preoperative PA radiograph the amount of narrowing would allow the styloid to come within 2 mm of the ulnar deviated carpal bones, one may anticipate stylocarpal impingement. The treatment for this is a shortening of the ulna with a tension band, nonabsorbable sutures through drill holes, anchors, or other forms of fixation.

Summary

One of the critical requirements for this procedure to succeed is a functional TFCC structure. In rheumatoid arthritis or traumatic disruption of the DRUJ, the TFCC is unstable. If the TFCC can be reconstructed and DRUJ arthritis exists, this is the situation in which the hemiresection procedure excels. In the face of a normal DRUJ without arthritis, an ulnar shortening with a repair of the TFCC, if necessary, is the more appropriate procedure. The other caveat for this procedure to succeed is a careful preoperative plan to make sure stylocarpal impingement does not occur. The procedure does not restore stability in the unstable painful radioulnar joint; it simply substitutes a less painful instability. When correctly planned and performed the hemiresection interposition technique can be a good procedure in the arsenal of treatment for the DRUJ.

References

[1] Darrach W. Forward dislocation at the inferior radioulnar joint, with fracture of the lower third of the shaft of the radius. Ann Surg 1912;56:801.

[2] Bowers WH. Distal radioulnar joint arthroplasty: the hemiresection-interposition technique. J Hand Surg 1985;10A:169–78.

[3] Watson HK, Ryu J, Burgess R. Matched distal ulnar resection. J Hand Surg 1986;11A:812–7.

[4] Watson HK, Gabuzda GM. Match distal ulnar resection for post-traumatic disorders of the distal radioulnar joint. J Hand Surg 1992;17A:724–30.

[5] Bowers WH. The distal radioulnar joint. In: Green DP, editor. Operative hand surgery. 4th edition. New York: Churchill Livingstone; 1999. p. 986–1032.

[6] Bowers WH, Zelouf D. Treatment of chronic disorders of the distal radioulnar joint. In: Lichtman DM, editor. The wrist and its disorders. 2nd edition. Philadelphia: WB Saunders; 1997.

[7] Ekstam F, Engvist O, Wadin K. Results from resection of the distal end of the ulna after fractures of the lower end of the radius. Scand J Plast Reconstr Surg 1982;16:177–81.

[8] Bieber EJ, Linscheid RL, Dobyns JH, et al. Failed distal ulna resections. J Hand Surg 1988;13A: 193–200.

[9] Nolan WB, Eaton RG. A Darrach procedure for distal ulnar pathology derangements. Clin Orthop 1992;275:85–9.

[10] Rowland SA. Stabilization of the ulnar side of the rheumatoid wrist following radiocarpal arthroplasty and resection of the distal ulna. Orthop Trans 1982; 6:474.

[11] Debenedetto MR, Lubbers LM, Coleman CR. Long term results of the minimal resection Darrach procedure. J Hand Surg 1991;16A:445–50.

[12] Golcher JL, Hayes MO. Stabilization of the remaining ulna using one-half of the extensor carpi ulnaris tendon after resection of the distal ulna. Orthop Trans 1979;3:330–1.

[13] Kleinman WB, Greenberg JA. Salvage of the failed Darrach procedure. J Hand Surg 1995;20A: 951–8.

[14] Bell MJ, Hill RJ, McMurty RY. Ulnar impingement syndrome. J Bone Joint Surg 1985;67B:126–9.

[15] Minami A, Kaneda K, Iroga H. Hemiresection-interposition arthroplasty of the distal radioulnar joint associated with repair of triangular fibrocartilage complex lesions. J Hand Surg 1991;16A:1120–5.

[16] Wicks B, Fletcher D, Palmer AK. Failed Bowers procedure (HIT technique). Paper presented at the 45th Annual Meeting of the American Society for Hand Surgery; September 24–27, 1990; Toronto.

[17] Van Schoonhover J, Fernandez DL, Bowers WH, et al. Salvage of failed resection arthroplasties of the distal radioulnar joint using a new ulnar head prosthesis. J Hand Surg [Am] 2000;25(3):438–46.

[18] Imbriglia JE, Matthew D. Treatment of chronic post-traumatic dorsal subluxation of the distal ulna by hemiresection interpositional arthroplasty. J Hand Surg 1993;18A:899–907.

[19] Sauerbier M, Berger RA, Fujita M, et al. Radioulnar convergence after distal ulnar resection. Acta Orthop Scand 2003;74(4):420–8.

[20] Greenberg JA, Yanagida H, Wemer FU, et al. Wide excision of the distal ulna: biomechanical testing of a salvage procedure. J Hand Surg 2003;28A:105–10.

[21] Bernstein MA, Nagle DJ, Martinez A, et al. A comparison of combined arthroscopic triangular fibrocartilage complex debridement and arthroscopic wafer distal ulna resection versus arthroscopic triangular fibrocartilage complex debridement and ulnar shortening osteotomy for ulnocarpal abutment syndrome. J Arthroscopic Rel Surg 2004;20(4): 392–401.

[22] Ekenstam F. The anatomy of the distal radioulnar joint. Clin Orthop 1992;275:14–8.

[23] Kauer JMG. The distal radioulnar joint: anatomical and functional considerations. Clin Orthop 1992; 275:37–45.

[24] Bowers WH. The distal radioulnar joint. In: Green DP, editor. Operative hand surgery. 4th edition. New York: Churchill Livingstone; 1999. p. 988.

[25] Palmar AK, Glisson RR, Werner FW. Relationship between ulnar variance and triangular cartilage complex thickness. J Hand Surg 1984;9A:681–3.

[26] Palmar AK, Werner FW. Biomechanics of the distal radioulnar joint. Clin Orthop 1984;187:26–34.

[27] Palmar AK. Triangular fibrocartilage complex lesions: a classification. J Hand Surg 1989;14A: 594–606.

[28] Palmar AK, Werner FW. The triangular fibrocartilage complex of the wrist: anatomy and function. J Hand Surg 1981;6:153–61.

[29] Bowers WH. The distal radioulnar joint. In: Green DP, editor. Operative hand surgery. 4th edition. New York: Churchill Livingstone; 1999. p. 992.

[30] Mikic ZD. Detailed anatomy of the articular disc of the distal radioulnar joint. Clin Orthop 1989;245: 123–32.

[31] Mikic ZD, Some L, Somer T. Histologic structure of the articular disc of the human distal radioulnar joint. Clin Orthop 1992;275:29–36.

[32] Chidgey LK, Dell PC, Bittar E, et al. Tear patterns and collagen arrangement in the triangular fibrocartilage. J Hand Surg 1987;16A:1084–100.

[33] Taleisnik J. The ligaments of the wrist. J Hand Surg 1976;1:110–8.

[34] King GJ, McMurtry RY, Rubenstein JD, et al. Kinematics of the distal radioulnar joint. J Hand Surg 1986;11A:798–804.

[35] Werner FW, Palmar AK, Fortino MD, et al. Force transmission through the distal ulna: effect of ulnar variance, lunate fossa angulation, and radial and palmar tilt of the distal radius. J Hand Surg 1992; 17A:423–8.

[36] Mikic ZD. Age changes in the triangular fibrocartilage of the wrist joint. J Anat 1978;126: 367–84.

[37] Bowers WH. The distal radioulnar joint. In: Green DP, editor. Operative hand surgery. 4th edition. New York: Churchill Livingstone; 1999. p. 1021.

[38] Ruby LK, Frenez CC, Dell PC. The pronator quadratus interposition transfer. An adjunct to distal radioulnar joint resection arthroplasty. J Hand Surg 1996;21A:60–5.

[39] Dell PC. Distal radioulnar joint dysfunction. Hand Clin 1987;3(4):563–82.

[40] Adams BD. Distal radioulnar joint instability. AAOS Instr Course 1998;47:209–13.

Use of an Ulnar Head Endoprosthesis for Treatment of an Unstable Distal Ulnar Resection: Review of Mechanics, Indications, and Surgical Technique

Richard A. Berger, MD, PhD*, William P. Cooney III, MD

Mayo Clinic College of Medicine, 200 First Street SW, Rochester, MN 55905, USA

Arthrosis of the distal radioulnar joint (DRUJ) can occur as the result of inflammatory arthropathy, traumatic disruption of the articular surfaces of the ulnar head or sigmoid notch, traumatic disruption of the soft tissue constraints between the radius and ulna (leading to instability), infection, and developmental malformation of the radius or ulna (leading to altered joint mechanics of the DRUJ). Painful arthrosis of the DRUJ is a common problem that often leads to substantial disability from pain, weakness, and instability. After degenerative changes in the articular surfaces of the DRUJ have developed, surgical options are largely limited to salvage procedures because there are no known reliable procedures that can reconstitute the joint articular cartilage. Therefore, resection of one or both surfaces of the distal ulna has been the most popular surgical treatment [1–4]. This treatment can take several forms, such as complete resection of the ulnar head (Darrach [2]); partial resection of the distal joint surfaces (Feldon and colleagues [5]) or proximal joint surface (Bowers [1]) with or without soft tissue interposition [6]; or fusion of the distal radius and ulna, with creation of a proximal pseudarthrosis (Kapandji-Sauvé procedure [7–9]).

The most basic and time-honored method of resecting the arthritic surface of the DRUJ was introduced in 1912 by Darrach [2]; however, it was first mentioned by Moore 1880 in the American literature for fresh injuries and in the German literature by Lauenstein 1887 [10]. By convention, the term *Darrach resection* implies resection of the entire ulnar head. Although modifications of the technique have evolved, complications related to instability of the distal forearm resulting from loss of the ulnar head have remained and are presented as the principal detractor of this procedure [11–16]. Instability of the distal radius and wrist relative to the shortened ulna has been typically recognized as an anterior-posterior instability [11,13,17–21]. This instability secondary to ulna resection results in weakness of grip strength and torsional strength of the forearm. In addition, however, a convergence instability of the stump of the resected ulna (ulna impingement syndrome [12]) toward the metaphysis of the radius has been identified as a cause of progressive pain following Darrach resection or similar procedures.

Stuart and colleagues [21] reported that approximately 20% of the total constraint of the DRUJ is contributed by articular contact between the distal radius and ulna. Although not specifically proved in a laboratory setting, it is possible that some loss of stability following resection of the distal ulna results from loss of the "cam effect" of the DRUJ, which normally separates the radius and ulna. This separation may physiologically tense the interosseous membrane, which provides a stabilizing element for the forearm joint. Loss of the cam effect effectively relaxes the interosseous membrane, rendering it less effective in stabilizing the forearm joint. Resecting the distal ulna, in part or entirely, results in an enhanced tendency for convergence of the distal radius toward the ulna [12,15,16]. In clinical cases, there remains a strong necessity to resect the

* Corresponding author.

E-mail address: berger.richard@mayo.edu (R.A. Berger).

0749-0712/05/$ - see front matter © 2005 Elsevier Inc. All rights reserved.
doi:10.1016/j.hcl.2005.08.015

arthritic distal ulna because of the pain related to loss of the articular surfaces despite the instability and radioulnar bone convergence that may result [11,22–26]. The suggestion that a prosthetic replacement of the distal ulna is physiologically sound has been suggested by several studies of the DRUJ [20,27–35]. To provide a better alternative and to correct pain related to distal ulna resections, endoprostheses have recently been developed to replace the mechanical function of the ulnar head [33,34,36]. One of these devices, developed at the Mayo Clinic, consists of a titanium sprayed–cobalt metallic stem that inserts into the shaft of the ulna and a polished cobalt, chrome, metallic ulnar head. The latter has channels for provisional soft tissue attachments by way of sutures into the triangular fibrocartilage complex (TFCC) and the subsheath of the extensor carpi ulnaris (ECU) (Fig. 1).

Anatomy

Osseous

The bony anatomy of the DRUJ must be understood in the context of the entire forearm. Hagert [20] referred to the DRUJ as one part of the "forearm joint" to emphasize the interdependence of the DRUJ with the remainder of the forearm. The distal radius metaphysis and epiphysis expand in the medial-lateral dimension as the wrist is approached. The ulnar (medial) surface of the radius is essentially parallel with the diaphysis of the radius, and forms the foundation for the

sigmoid notch (see Fig. 1). The sigmoid notch is a shallow, variable-sized concavity lined with hyaline cartilage that articulates with the ulnar head. The radius of curvature of the sigmoid notch is larger than the articular surface of the ulnar head (Fig. 2). The sigmoid notch is shaped like a rectangle when viewed "en face" from the medial surface but possesses a concavity in the anterior-posterior direction. The dorsal and palmar margins of the sigmoid notch serve as respective attachment surfaces for the dorsal and palmar radioulnar ligaments and the dorsal and palmar aspects of the DRUJ capsule. The shape of the sigmoid notch can be different, as observed by af Ekenstam and Hagert [37]. These investigators measured the curvature of the sigmoid notch, with an arch of 47° to 80° and a radius that averaged 15 mm in diameter (range, 12–28 mm). DeSmet and Fabry [38] reported on different morphologies of the sigmoid notch. They randomly evaluated 100 posteroanterior (PA) radiographs of the wrist and concluded that in an ulna-plus wrist, there is a hemispheric-shaped sigmoid fossa, whereas in the ulna-minus wrist, the shape of the notch is conic. In the ulna-neutral wrist, it is usually cylindric and sometimes conic.

The distal end of the ulna is complex in shape, composed of the ulnar neck, ulnar head, and ulnar styloid process (Fig. 3). The ulnar neck represents the distal metaphysis of the ulna and serves as an attachment of the palmar and dorsal regions of the DRUJ capsule. The neck also represents the transition between the periosteum-covered

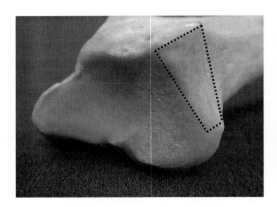

Fig. 1. Oblique view of the distal radius demonstrating the location of the sigmoid notch. The shape and orientation of the sigmoid notch is highly variable. (Courtesy of Mayo Clinic College of Medicine, Rochester, MN; with permission.)

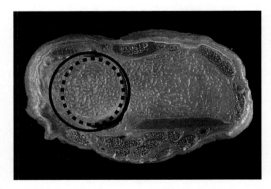

Fig. 2. Cross-sectional view of the DRUJ demonstrating the difference in radius of curvature of the sigmoid notch (*solid line*) and the ulnar head (*dotted line*). This difference in curvature allows a combination of rotation and translation, or a gliding motion, between the distal radius and ulna. (Courtesy of Mayo Clinic College of Medicine, Rochester, MN; with permission.)

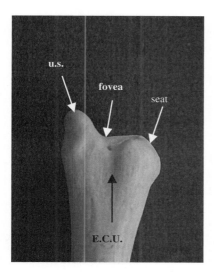

Fig. 3. Posterior view of an ulnar head. u.s., ulnar styloid process; E.C.U., groove for the tendon of the extensor carpi ulnaris. (Courtesy of Mayo Clinic College of Medicine, Rochester, MN; with permission.)

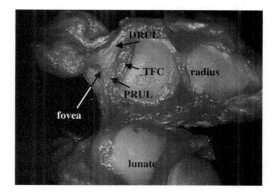

Fig. 4. Dissection of a cadaver wrist from a distal perspective, with the proximal row flexed maximally. DRUL, dorsal radioulnar ligament; PRUL, palmar radioulnar ligament; TFC, triangular fibrocartilage. (Courtesy of Mayo Clinic College of Medicine, Rochester, MN; with permission.)

diaphysis and the hyaline cartilage–covered ulna head. The head of the ulna is a hemicylindric enlargement of the distal end of the ulna, covered by hyaline cartilage on its distal, dorsal, medial, and palmar surfaces. The articular surface facing the sigmoid notch is oriented such that it is roughly parallel with the inclination of the sigmoid notch. Distally, the dome of the ulnar head is slightly convex and mostly covered in articular cartilage. The ulnar styloid process is a longitudinally oriented distal projection of the posterior cortex of the ulna. It is of variable length, but usually 4 to 6 mm. At the base of the styloid process, where it joins the dome of the ulnar head, there is a non-cartilage–covered area called the fovea that serves as the insertion site for a number of important ligaments. Between the posterior cylindric articular surface of the ulnar head and the styloid process is the groove for the tendon of ECU.

Ligamentous

The anatomy of the soft tissues supporting of the DRUJ is complex [21,24,28,30,37,39–42]. At the center is the TFCC. It is located to function as a collateral ligament system, essentially draped over the distal end of the ulna [41], and composed of several components (Fig. 4) [42–44]. At the center of the ligamentous complex is the triangular fibrocartilage (TFC). This structure forms an almost equilateral triangle that is attached to the radius along the distal edge and lunate fossa of the distal radius and to the prestyloid recess, the ulnar extent of the TFC. The TFC has a thickness that is proportional to the ulnar variance (ie, the degree of length discrepancy between the distal radius and ulna). Negative ulnar variance, indicating an ulna shorter than the radius, is associated with a thicker TFC. Conversely, a positive ulnar variance is associated with a progressively thinner TFC [20].

The dorsal and palmar radioulnar ligaments are closely integrated with the dorsal and palmar margins of the TFC, but progressively form clearly discrete, independent structures proximally (see Fig. 4) [37,40,44,45]. The dorsal radioulnar ligament originates at the dorsal margin of the sigmoid notch and courses obliquely across the ulnar head to insert into the fovea. The most superficial fibers of the dorsal radioulnar ligament split to contribute to the formation of the ECU tendon subsheath, an important secondary stabilizer of the DRUJ. Radially, the dorsal radioulnar ligament is reinforced by arcuate fibers from the ulnar margin of the distal radius metaphysis. The palmar radioulnar ligament also originates radially along the palmar margin of the sigmoid notch of the radius and courses obliquely and dorsally to insert at the fovea of the distal ulna. It gives rise to the ulnocarpal ligaments. The obliquity of the palmar and dorsal radioulnar ligaments results in a convergence to form a conjoined ligament. The conjoined ligament attaches to the ulna at the fovea and then inserts again along a variable length of the ulnar styloid process. If the band between the foveal and styloid attachments of the conjoined ligament is free from continuous attachment to the ulna, then the space between the ulna and the conjoined ligament forms what has been referred to as the "ligamentum subcruentum" [41]. With resection of the distal ulna, the continuity of these structures must be maintained to preserve elements of distal ulnar stability. Knowledge of ligament anatomy is essential in consideration of prosthetic replacement of the distal ulna. Retaining normal ligamentous anatomy or reconstruction of support ligaments is critical to the stability of an ulnar head prosthesis.

Mechanics

Kinematics

Because of the rigid-body nature of the radius and ulna, the kinematics of the DRUJ must be considered as only one aspect of forearm kinematics [17,19,20,28,32,37,44]. As such, motion generated at the proximal radioulnar joint is reflected in motion at the DRUJ, and vice versa. It must also be remembered that because of this rigid-body relationship, instability or abnormal kinematics at the proximal radioulnar joint (eg, radial head excision) is reflected in abnormal motion at the DRUJ. Instability and abnormal kinematics (secondary to bone loss of distal ulnar and its support ligaments) affect forearm rotation, alignment, and stability.

Overall, the kinematics of the forearm are rotational, with the mobile segment being the radius rotating about the fixed element, the ulna [28]. Studies have shown that as a generalization, rotation of the forearm occurs about an axis rotation passing through the radial head proximally and the ulnar head (ulnar fovea) distally (Fig. 5). This axis could be fixed if rotation was the only displacement mode, but this would require essentially a "log roll" of the radius about the ulna. Rather, a pivoting motion is found, occurring at the pivot of the proximal radioulnar joint and extending along the rotational forearm axion to the DRUJ. This pivoting motion results in a combination of rotation and translation through the DRUJ (see Fig. 5B) [28,30,44]. This observation of forearm kinematics is evidenced by a shift in the position of the plane of intersection of the axis of rotation and the cortex of the ulnar head such that the axis shifts anteriorly

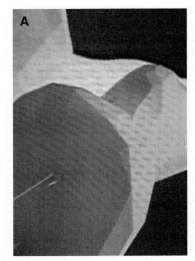

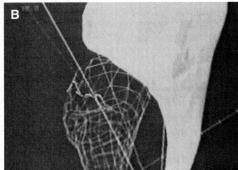

Fig. 5. Computer-generated images obtained from CT examination of a forearm with superimposed axis of forearm rotation obtained from a kinematic study using a magnetic tracking system. (*A*) View of the radial head, showing the penetration of the forearm axis of rotation coincident with the geometric center of the radial head. (*B*) View of the ulnar head (*grid*) and radius (*solid*), with the axis of rotation passing through the ulnar head. The axis of rotation translates anteriorly and posteriorly during forearm pronation and supination, respectively, as evidenced by the "trail" marked at the penetration point of the axis in the ulnar head.

during pronation and posteriorly during supination. The magnitude of this shift approaches 5 mm under normal circumstances and is allowed by the differences in radii of curvature of the ulnar head and the sigmoid notch. The limits of translation are principally constrained by soft tissues, as described later. An ulnar head prosthesis must duplicate the normal kinematics to restore full forearm rotation with a proper axis of rotation.

Stability analyses

The contribution to stability of the DRUJ has been studied in several investigations, each looking at different aspects of the question. af Eckenstam and Hagert [37] evaluated the effects of sectioning the dorsal and palmar radioulnar ligaments on tendencies to subluxation of the DRUJ. They discovered that the dorsal radioulnar ligament provides the greatest constraint against dorsal subluxation of the radius relative to the ulna in supination. Conversely, the palmar radioulnar ligament contributed most against dorsal subluxation of the radius relative to the ulna in pronation. Schuind and colleagues [44] took a different tack and evaluated the degree of strain in the dorsal and palmar radioulnar ligaments relative to forearm position. They discovered that the dorsal radioulnar ligament underwent maximal strain during pronation and the palmar radioulnar ligament underwent maximal strain during supination.

Stuart and coworkers [21] studied the effects of sectioning the dorsal and palmar radioulnar ligaments, the ulnocarpal ligaments, the interosseous membrane, and the ECU tendon subsheath on constraints against displacement in neutral, midpronation, and midsupination. This study showed that the palmar radioulnar ligament was the principle constraint against palmar displacement of the radius relative to the ulna (ie, dorsal displacement of the distal ulna). The interosseous membrane provided substantially less constraints, and the ulnocarpal ligaments and tendon subsheath complexes provided negligible constraint. Constraints against dorsal displacement of the radius relative to the ulna are, in general, more complex, involving variable contributions from the dorsal radioulnar ligament and the interosseous membrane. A critical finding was the residual constraint level after all soft tissues were compromised, ranging from 20% to 30%. This residual constraint was attributed to the articular contact between the ulnar head and the sigmoid notch. Absence of the ulnar head reduced stability of the DRUJ at a minimum of 30%. Haugstvedt and colleagues [46] studied the effects of sectioning the foveal and styloid insertions of the TFCC relative to forearm position. This study showed that a significantly greater degree of loss of constraint was found with division of the foveal or styloid attachments of the TFCC compared with the isolated division of the dorsal and palmar radioulnar ligaments. This phenomenon was

independent of forearm position and there was no statistical difference between foveal or styloid disruption. Finally, a recent laboratory study emphasized the importance of the palmar and dorsal DRUJ capsule as a stabilizer in the extremes of supination and pronation, respectively [47]. Restoration of the soft tissue constraints (back to the distal ulna) is therefore as important as preservation or replacement of the ulnar head. Prosthetic replacement of the distal ulna must consider the important restoration of the TFC, ECU subsheath, and dorsal and palmar radioulnar ligaments.

Kinetics

Kinetic studies have demonstrated that the magnitude of axially (longitudinally) transmitted forces across the ulnocarpal joint [48] is approximately 20% of the load transmitted across the wrist [25]. This load is proportionately increased with different positions of the wrist and forearm. During wrist ulnar deviation, the centroid of muscle force is shifted ulnarly, resulting in a relative unloading of the radiocarpal joint reactive force and an increase in ulnocarpal contact force. In addition, pathologic conditions that result in a more distal projection of the ulna relative to the radius result in increased ulnocarpal contact forces. Examples of these include developmental positive variance of the ulna and shortening of the radius from conditions such as distal radius fractures or radial head resection. Finally, due to the pivot phenomenon resulting in relative positive ulnar variance in forearm pronation described previously, pronation of the forearm leads to progressively larger ulnocarpal contact forces compared with supination.

Etiology of arthrosis

Inflammatory arthritis, particularly rheumatoid arthritis, is a clear cause of pain and disability of the DRUJ [22] and no doubt stems from an early pannus involvement of the DRUJ and ulnocarpal joint due to the high degree of vascularity in this region. Inflammatory arthritis results in destruction of the articular surfaces of the ulnar head and the sigmoid notch, with simultaneous loss of soft tissue integrity, leading to further instability and pain. Loss of soft tissue stability leads to the commonly observed condition known as caput ulnae syndrome [49,50]. Even when the inflammatory phase of the disease is quiescent, it is usual for patients who have rheumatoid arthritis to continue to have problems associated with residual degenerative disease and instability.

Post-traumatic causes for degenerative arthritis of the DRUJ largely result from a malunited Colles' fracture involving the sigmoid notch of the distal radius [23,25]. Arthritis of the DRUJ is the second most common complication of Colles' fracture [23], especially when considering fractures involving the articular surface of the sigmoid notch proper. These fractures can split the sigmoid notch into dorsal and palmar fragments, not only creating articular surface incongruities but also creating unstable avulsion fractures of the radial attachments of the dorsal and palmar radioulnar ligaments. Even in the face of an anatomic reduction and union of the distal radius, the initial energy of injury causing a fracture may lead to chondrolysis and degenerative arthritis of the DRUJ. A second class of post-traumatic change results from injuries to the soft tissues that stabilize the DRUJ, especially TFC tears or ulnar styloid fractures. Such injuries may lead to chronic instability. Chronic instability over time leads to destruction of the articular surfaces of the DRUJ.

The final category of patients presenting with definite degenerative changes in the DRUJ is idiopathic, resulting from congenital or developmental abnormalities of the geometry of the joint surfaces (eg, Madelung's deformity) or laxity of the soft tissues.

Diagnosis

Although radiographs may show substantial arthritic changes in the surfaces of the DRUJ, there may be a period of relative quiescence of symptoms in the patient who has arthrosis of the DRUJ. After symptoms appear, the detrimental effect on forearm function usually forces the patient to seek medical evaluation. The diagnosis of arthritis at the DRUJ is relatively straightforward. The patient presents with symptoms of pain in the region of the DRUJ, exacerbated with activity. Pain increases with gripping and resisted rotation of the forearm and is described as having an aching quality with sharp exacerbations. Swelling may be a feature. When combined with increased warmth, these findings of pain and swelling should alert the clinician to the possibility of the presence of degenerative or inflammatory arthritis of the DRUJ.

Findings on physical examination typically include tenderness about the ulnar head. There may be crepitance with forearm rotation. The patient may report an increase in discomfort with direct compression of the ulna against the radius at the level of the DRUJ, especially while rotating the forearm. Dorsal or palmar translation of the radius relative to the ulna, with or without a palpable or audible "click," may be present. Care should be taken to compare the findings on the symptomatic side to the contralateral wrist and forearms. Pain may also be present at the extremes of forearm pronation and supination, especially in early arthritis. Prominence of the ulna should be assessed in all forearm positions and compared with the contralateral DRUJ. The appearance of a prominent ulnar head may indicate (1) a subluxated DRUJ secondary to TFC or dorsal/palmar radioulnar ligament injury or (2) disruption of the ulnocarpal ligaments leading to ulnocarpal supination. A simple maneuver may help to clarify this differential diagnosis: one can simply exert a dorsally directed force on the pisiform. If the prominent ulnar head recedes, then it is likely due to ulnocarpal supination. If the ulna head remains displaced, then a DRUJ subluxation or dislocation is present.

Radiographic assessment

Standard PA and lateral radiographs (Fig. 6) are typically all that are needed to confirm the status of the DRUJ joint. It is critical, however, that these radiographs be obtained in a standard

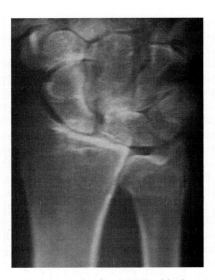

Fig. 6. PA radiograph of a DRUJ with degenerative joint disease.

fashion to minimize the effects of forearm rotation. The PA radiograph is taken with the x-ray source directly centered over the DRUJ, with the shoulder laterally abducted 90°, the elbow flexed 90°, and the palm flat on the x-ray cassette in neutral rotation. The lateral radiograph is obtained with the patient's shoulder in neutral adduction such that the arm is at his or her side, the elbow is flexed 90°, and the ulnar border of the hand is resting on the x-ray cassette in neutral flexion/extension. If there is any concern about the specific status of the DRUJ articular surfaces, such as geometry, incongruity, or orientation, then CT (Fig. 7) scans offer the most definitive test. CT offers the advantage of obtaining simultaneous comparative axial images (to show dorsal or palmar instability) and adds the possibility of obtaining images in multiple positions of forearm rotation. In addition, imaging of the contralateral DRUJ offers an excellent opportunity for comparisons.

Conservative management

Unless some feature of presentation is worrisome, such as pending tendon rupture, it is best to initiate and strongly persist with conservative measures on all patients who have arthrosis of DRUJ. As an example, after Colles' fracture, it may take 1 year for the DRUJ to become asymptomatic. The conservative measures often include the use of nonsteroidal anti-inflammatory

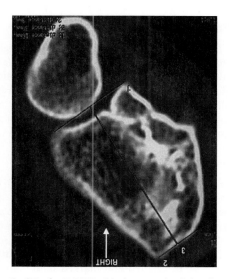

Fig. 7. CT of a DRUJ with degenerative joint disease.

drugs, forearm splints (including the elbow and wrist), the option of corticosteroid injections into the DRUJ, and activity modification. In acute and subacute cases of DRUJ injury, a supportive ulnar gutter splint or a "pisiform" lift splint to correct carpal supination may be beneficial. The optimum form of splinting of the DRUJ should include immobilization of the elbow.

Rationale for development of an ulnar head implant

The rationale for development of an ulnar head replacement is based on the mechanical concept of the forearm joint. The anatomy, kinematics, and kinetics described earlier point to the importance of this concept. Although relief from pain at the DRUJ may be gained by simply resecting the distal ulna, in a very real way, this disrupts the stability of the entire forearm and often leads to forearm instability. This result may not be a significant problem in patients who lead low-demand lives, but in active individuals, distal ulnar resection results in substantial reduction in stability, torque strength, and decreased upper-limb function. It frequently leads to painful impingement of the stump of the ulna during active use [12]. This painful phenomenon has been shown to be due to a convergence instability of the stump of the ulna against the distal radius. Reports on the use of soft tissues to stabilize the stump of the ulna (Fig. 8) have questionable success. Surgical procedures such as interposition of the pronator quadratus, tenodesis with the flexor carpi ulnaris and ECU tendons [18,51], and lengthening of the ulna [13] have not had great success in the authors' experience. None have been shown to restore forearm stability or prevent impingement [14]. Kapandji [8] attempted to solve the problem imposed by Darrach resections by performing arthrodesis of the ulnar head to the sigmoid notch of the radius and creating a pseudarthrosis at the level of the ulnar neck. It is unfortunate that this procedure has the same predisposition for convergence instability as the Darrach resection.

Indications for hemiprosthetic replacement of the distal ulna

There are primary and secondary indications to consider with ulnar head replacement. Primary indications include (1) comminuted distal ulna

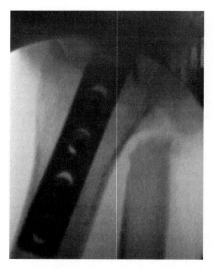

Fig. 8. PA radiograph of a wrist following a Darrach resection demonstrating the convergence of the distal radius toward the osteotomized distal ulna.

fracture, (2) Galeazzi variants of distal radius and distal ulnar fractures, (3), intraoperative evidence of excessive instability of the forearm joint following distal ulnar resection, and (4) primary inflammatory (rheumatoid) arthritis. In rheumatoid arthritis, arthritic changes with loss of joint cartilage but no gross bone loss within the DRUJ should be present to recommend distal ulna replacement. In many, if not most cases of carpal translation, a distal ulna prosthesis should be considered. It is also possible to correct carpal supination by combining a distal ulna prosthesis with a ligament soft tissue stabilization such as the Linscheid-Hui procedure [52].

Secondary indications for distal ulna replacement include (1) failure of a previous resection arthroplasty of the DRUJ (eg, Darrach resection or Bower's procedure); (2) failed silicone ulna head replacement [53,54]; and (3) failed DRUJ stabilization procedures. Ulna head replacement is also indicated to correct radiographic evidence of convergence instability following ulnar head resection (Darrach procedure) or one of its variations.

Contraindications for hemiprosthetic implantation

General contraindications for implantation of an ulnar head hemiprosthesis are the same as for other joint implants: infection, current or past history of inadequate soft tissues to provide a stable joint, regional neurologic pain dysfunction, and severe axial forearm instability (the Essex Lopresti lesion), unless the radial head is also replaced.

Contraindications may also be related to specific features of the radius and ulna and the soft tissue stabilizers of the forearm. Regarding features of the radius, a primary contraindication for implantation of an ulnar head hemiprosthesis is a radius malunion resulting in malalignment of the sigmoid notch relative to the radius. A corrective osteotomy of the radius should be considered before performing a distal ulnar prosthetic replacement. Similarly, previous pathology or trauma to the distal ulnar diaphysis (previous plate fixation) may create a potential difficulty for passing and securing the stem of the prosthesis within the medullary canal of the distal ulna.

Malunion of the metaphysis and diaphysis of the radius or ulna should be corrected before or simultaneously with ulna head replacement. Metabolic conditions of the ulna (eg, advanced osteoporosis) resulting in mechanically inferior bone stock should be considered a relative contraindication for implantation. Finally, soft tissue injuries resulting in loss of competence of the interosseous membrane and ligaments at the DRUJ should be considered a contraindication unless specific measures can be taken at the time of ulnar head implantation to stabilize the forearm joint and DRUJ (eg, Adams procedure [45] or Linscheid-Hui procedures to restore ligament support [52]).

Surgical technique

The following is a description of the surgical technique specific for the Avanta U-Head (Avanta Orthopedics, New York, New York) ulnar head endoprosthesis. The authors recognize the availability of other ulnar head implant systems and suggest careful consultation of the surgical technique guides specific for those systems before use.

Patient preparation

Radiographic templates may be used to determine the preferred size of the ulnar stem and ulnar head (Fig. 9), using the diseased wrist and normal wrist and forearm as a guide. Preoperative antibiotics are typically administered before incision. The patient is placed supine on the operating table. The designated and marked limb (surgical site) is prepped and draped in a sterile fashion.

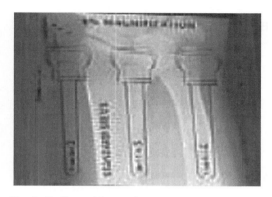

Fig. 9. Radiographic templates are necessary to determine the proper size of ulna head implant. (Courtesy of Avanta Orthopedics, Small Bone Innovations, New York, NY; with permission.)

Axillary block anesthesia is preferred, although general anesthesia is certainly acceptable. The extremity is exsanguinated with an Esmarch bandage and an upper-arm tourniquet is inflated.

Primary implantation

A dorsal-ulnar or dorsal longitudinal incision is made, centered over the head of the distal ulna (Fig. 10A, B). Soft tissue flaps are elevated, and dorsal sensory branches of ulnar nerve are identified and protected. The extensor retinaculum is divided through the fifth extensor compartment, allowing translocation of the extensor digiti minimi tendon (see Fig. 10C). An alternate approach is through a midmedial incision, developing a plane between the tendons of the extensor and flexor carpi ulnaris muscles. The capsule is released dorsally off the ulna in line with the proximal periosteum and deep to the ECU subsheath, which is reflected ulnarly (see Fig. 10D). The head of the ulna is exposed, with care taken to preserve the radial attachment of the TFCC. The TFCC is released at the fovea of the ulnar styloid or, alternatively, the ulnar styloid is osteotomized and left in continuity with the TFC.

A resection guide is used to mark the site of distal ulna resection, whereby the tab of the guide is placed firmly in the fovea and the osteotomy is marked for the size of prosthesis templated (see Fig. 10E, F). The authors recommending making a more conservative osteotomy (leaving more ulnar length) when any question about precision of osteotomy length or orientation exists. The osteotomy can always be revised before implant placement. Holman elevators are used to protect the soft tissues, and an oscillating saw is used to divide the ulna at the marked site (see Fig. 10G). The ulna head is removed.

The intramedullary canal of the ulna is then entered with an awl (see Fig. 10H) and broached to the correct diameter. The broach length matches the ulna stem length. The size of broach is based on the size determined by preoperative templates and intraoperative assessment. It is necessary to broach up and down (proximal then distal) and not to simply impact the broach.

The trial ulna stem is inserted and gently tapped into place (see Fig. 10I). If it is difficult to insert, then further broaching is required.

The trial ulna head is placed over the trial ulnar stem (see Fig. 10J). Care is taken to not use the definitive stem or ulnar head because the distal post of the proximal component (the Morris taper on the head–stem junction) will not allow for later separation. Radiographs (PA and lateral) are taken to judge proper length and alignment. To truly judge the length of the implant relative to the subchondral cortical line of the lunate fossa (as an estimate of ulnar implant variance), the forearm can be rotated under live fluoroscopy until the distal surface of the implant appears as an absolute straight line. This view represents the true PA projection of the implant. Stability of the forearm and the DRUJ are assessed, and correct alignment of the ulnar head within the sigmoid fossa is confirmed. There should be good dorsal-palmar stability at this stage. If radiographic alignment and clinical appearance and stability are present, then the definitive ulnar stem is inserted with the supplied tap, with care taken not to deform the Morris taper of the proximal stem during impaction. One must avoid direct metal hammer contact on the Morris taper. The use of bone cement should be considered in patients who have rheumatoid arthritis, significant osteoporosis, or a coexisting complete wrist arthrodesis and under circumstances where it is not possible to complete an ulnar shaft broaching with a larger size broach after completing a broach with a smaller size. In this last circumstance, the smaller size stem is placed and the void created by the partial broaching with the larger broach is filled with cement.

With the stem fully inserted, attention is now directed to soft tissue repair. The ulnar head has two holes for soft tissue attachment (see Fig. 10K). A number 0 or 2.0 polyfibril suture is placed through the ulnar border of the TFC and attached to the ulnar head (locking suture). A second suture is placed within the ECU subsheath

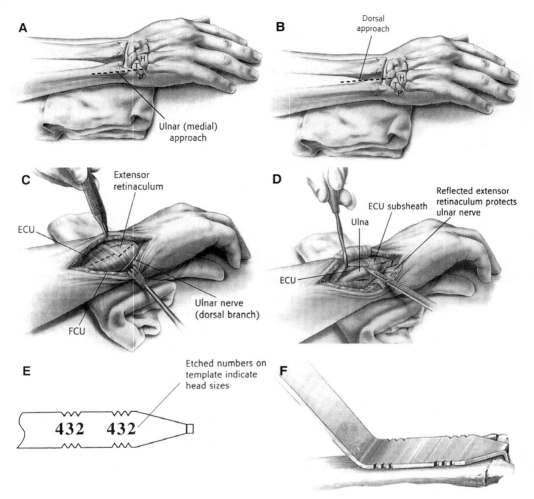

Fig. 10. (*A*) Ulnar skin incision, between the extensor and flexor carpi ulnaris tendons. (*B*) Dorsoulnar skin incision, radial to the tendon of ECU. (*C*) Exposure of the extensor retinaculum. The fifth extensor compartment is incised, allowing translocation of the tendon of extensor digiti minimi. The dorsal sensory branch of the ulnar nerve should be protected to avoid injury. (*D*) The head of the ulna is exposed subperiosteally, including division of the foveal attachment of the TFCC. Efforts are made to preserve the ECU tendon subsheath. (*E*) The osteotomy cutting guide has two sets of markings: the set nearest the tab is for primary implants and the set nearest the handle is for revision implants requiring an extension collar. (*F*) The tab of the osteotomy cutting guide is placed in the foveal recess at the base of the ulnar styloid process. (*G*) The ulnar osteotomy is completed, with appropriate soft tissue protection. (*H*) After removing the ulnar head, the medullary canal of the distal ulnar is broached to the proper size for the stem size templated. (*I*) A trial stem implant is advanced into the broached distal ulna with a tamp until the collar rests on the cut end of the ulna. (*J*) The proper head trial is placed on the stem, and the positioning of the implant is checked with intraoperative fluoroscopy. (*K*) After removal of the trial implants, two lengths of 2-0 braided nonresorbable suture are placed in the TFCC: one in the foveal attachment tissue and the other in the ECU tendon subsheath. (*L*) The foveal suture is advanced through the distal holes of the implant head, and the ECU subsheath sutures are advanced through the side holes. (*M*) The head is advanced onto the implant stem and rotated such that the sutures are just dorsal to the midposterior cortex, which is the same surface of the ulna as the posterior cortex of the olecranon. (*N*) The same procedure is followed for revision implants, with the additional step of trial fitting an extension collar. FCU, flexor carpi ulnaris; H, hamate; T, triquetrum; P, pisiform. (Courtesy of Avanta Orthopedics, Small Bone Innovations, New York, NY; with permission.)

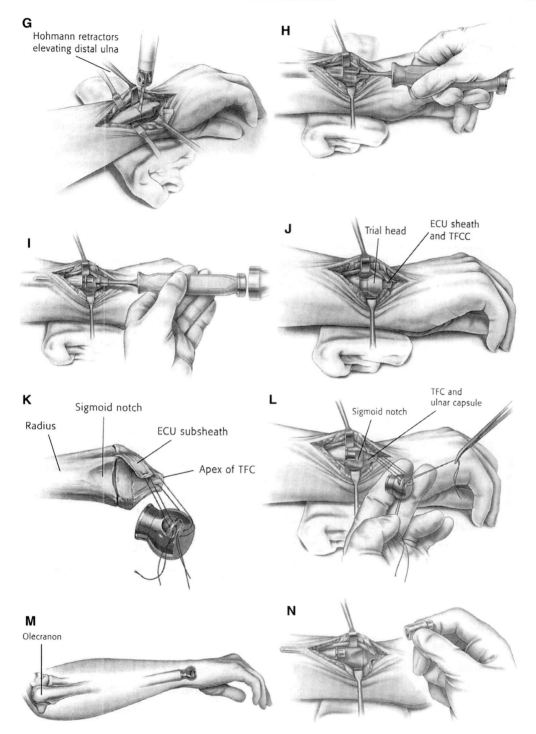

Fig. 10 *(continued)*

and through the second pair of holes in the ulnar head (see Fig. 10L).

The ulnar head is articulated onto the Morris taper of the proximal prosthesis stem and firmly tapped in place. The suture holes on the ulnar head must align with the true posterior cortex of the ulna or be rotated just dorsal to this true posterior position (see Fig. 10M). This positioning places the sutures in alignment with the ECU tendon and subsheath and minimizes confusion created by the rotating forearm. The ulnar head sutures are now tightened firmly in place. The forearm position should be the midposition (neutral pronation-supination). The dorsal DRUJ capsule is closed with the forearm in neutral rotation. The extensor retinaculum of the fifth compartment is closed after relocating the extensor digit minimi tendon, after which the subcutaneous tissues and skin are closed, over a suction drain if necessary.

The forearm is immobilized in midrotation to supination depending on DRUJ stability. Forearm position is maintained in a long-arm "sugar tong" placed splint. A long-arm cast (midrotation to forearm supination) is placed at 48 hours and left in place for 4 to 5 weeks.

Revision procedure

For revision procedures, preoperative templating using the extended prosthesis templates and normal wrist for comparison is an important first step in choosing ulnar head replacement with the extended collar. The template should overlay the PA radiograph to determine the correct size of stem, level of resection of the distal ulna, and level of revision and ulnar head.

Previous incisions (dorsal or ulnar) are incised, starting in scar-free tissue proximally and working distally. The dorsal ulnar cutaneous nerves are identified.

The extensor retinaculum is reflected as described earlier between the ECU and extensor digiti minimi. The capsule is usually scarred from previous surgery. It should now be released on the dorsal-ulnar aspect of the distal radius or directly ulnarly—but not directly dorsal—to allow for later closure of the DRUJ "compartment." A capsular compartment should be formed as the capsule is reflected.

The proximal ulna is identified and subperiosteal exposure is performed. Distally, the sigmoid notch is freed of scar tissue, and a DRUJ compartment consisting of the dorsal and volar

capsule, TFC (distally), ECU subsheath, and dorsal and volar DRUJ ligaments is created to receive and support the distal ulna prosthesis.

The alignment guide (see Fig. 10E) is used to determine the level of resection of the distal ulna. A new proximal ulna level of resection is created as measured. The ulna intramedullary canal is now broached. The trial stem (with extended collar) is inserted and the trial ulnar head is tapped into place (see Fig. 10N). Stability and appropriate length are examined clinically and radiographically. If correct, then the definitive stem with the extended collar is inserted as described earlier. Care is again taken in the soft tissue repair to the ulnar head. The soft tissues are attached first to the ulnar head. The ulnar head is articulated to the Morris taper and tapped into place, and the sutures are tightened. ECU subsheath and TFCC suture to the ulna head is performed before head articulation to the Morris taper. The capsule is closed and the stability of the prosthesis is checked again during forearm rotation. The ulnar alignment and length are checked using biplanar radiographs.

The U-Head should be attached to the TFC, ECU subsheath, and dorsal capsule with 0 or 2.0 polyfilament sutures. A firm capsule closure is completed with an interlocking stitch, with the forearm in neutral pronation-supination. If instability of the prosthesis is noted at the time of trial prosthesis insertion, then ligament support augmentation may be necessary.

Special circumstances

Rheumatoid arthritis

In the rheumatoid patient, use of bone cement is recommended when inserting the ulnar head prosthesis. Bone cement is also recommended if there is an associated total wrist fusion or if there was a prior silicone distal ulna. Careful preservation of capsule and TFC is necessary to provide good soft tissue reconstruction of the DRUJ. For revision of failed distal ulna resection, proper length of prosthesis is necessary, along with soft tissue repair or reconstruction. A prosthesis placement with slight negative ulnar variance is preferred over a positive ulna variance. For ligament reconstruction, the authors have used the flexor carpi ulnaris (Hui-Linscheid procedure [52,55]) and the palmaris longus (Adams procedure variation [43,45]) to help stabilize the joint. In both

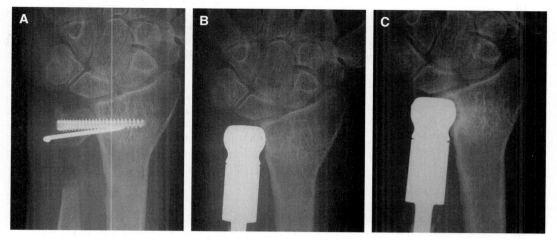

Fig. 11. (*A*) PA radiograph of a patient who underwent a Kapandji-Sauvé procedure. (*B*) PA radiograph of same patient following revision to an ulnar head implant arthroplasty. (*C*) Because the subchondral bone is compromised in the fusion process, subsequent implantation of a hemiarthroplasty may lead to subsidence of the implant into the radial metaphysis. (Courtesy of Mayo Clinic College of Medicine, Rochester, MN; with permission.)

procedures, the tendon is looped around the neck of the implant and is secured.

The authors have "freshened" the sigmoid fossa with a burr when it is shallow or scarred, with good clinical outcomes. Deepening the sigmoid fossa may be necessary if it is flat, if it is partially arthritic, and when instability of the DRUJ is a concern. If there is significant (complete) arthritic deterioration of the sigmoid fossa, then ulnar head replacement may not be indicated.

After ulnar head prosthetic replacement, a period of forearm and wrist immobilization is necessary to allow for soft tissue capsule healing and healing of the TFC and ECU subsheath. The forearm postoperatively is placed in midrotation (preferred) or supination (for revision procedures with ligament augmentation). A long-arm cast is used for 4 weeks, followed by a Munster brace (elbow flexion-extension allowed) for a further 4 weeks. The patient can be allowed out of the brace for gentle assisted forearm rotation. At 8 weeks, an ulnar gutter splint (elbow free) may also be used, with gradual weaning from the splint over 4 weeks. Active assisted motion is increased, and forearm and wrist strengthening are started. Patients are allowed to return to light-duty work at 8 weeks. Sports activities such as bowling, tennis, golf, waterskiing or downhill skiing are not

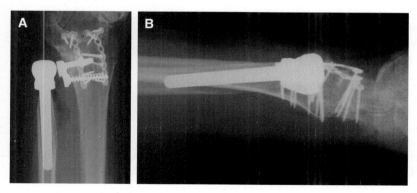

Fig. 12. PA (*A*) and lateral (*B*) radiographs of a wrist following implantation of a sigmoid notch arthroplasty component, matched to the ulnar head implant. (Courtesy of Mayo Clinic College of Medicine, Rochester, MN; with permission.)

allowed. If there is difficulty regaining forearm rotation, then a static-assist forearm splint is initiated under hand-therapist control.

Revision of a failed Kapandji-Sauvé procedure

The authors have treated the painful, unstable forearm resulting from a Kapandji-Sauvé procedure in the same manner as a revision ulnar head implantation. The ulnar head and associated hardware is resected, leaving the previous sigmoid notch exposed as a flat surface of cancellous bone. This bone is easily contoured to a shallow concavity with a burr, and a revision stem implant is placed as described earlier. The ulnar head implant is placed using standard provisional soft tissue fixation, also as described earlier (Fig. 11A, B).

Because the subchondral bone of the sigmoid notch is typically removed during the Kapandji-Sauvé procedure, there may be evidence of chronic convergence subsidence of the implant into the radial epiphysis, potentially undermining the mechanical integrity of the subchondral bone of the lunate fossa (see Fig. 11C). If convergence subsidence is believed to be a real threat, then revision bone grafting could be performed, although this has not been necessary in the authors' patients to date. In addition, this complication would be an indication for use of a recently developed sigmoid notch implant (Fig. 12).

Residual instability following ulnar head implant arthroplasty

Although residual instability following ulnar head implant arthroplasty has rarely been a clinically relevant problem, it has occurred and has required the development of some unique solutions. First, the underlying cause of the instability must be determined (this is where the contralateral radiographs obtained in the preoperative assessment can be valuable). If the patient has a malformed distal radius resulting from trauma (malunited Colles' fracture) of a developmental abnormality in the normal alignment of the radius, then this must be corrected through an osteotomy before any soft tissue stabilization procedures are contemplated (Fig. 13). A deficient sigmoid notch may also be the cause of residual instability and can be assessed with bilateral CT scans. The artifact from the metal of the implant can be minimized with modern radiographic technical protocols.

If the orientation of the sigmoid notch is acceptable, then one can assume that the instability is due to soft tissue deficiencies. The first step is to verify that the DRUJ can be manually reduced. If it is difficult to achieve a congruent reduction, then one should be suspicious of soft tissue interposition within the DRUJ. If it is reducible, then plans for soft tissue reconstruction can be contemplated. It must be remembered that the sutures initially placed during implantation of the device were meant for provisional fixation of the TFCC to the device. This and the capsular closure should produce what is essentially a soft tissue socket to contain the ulnar head. The importance of the joint capsule cannot be overemphasized. As such, residual instability should

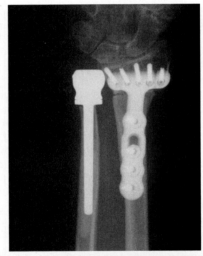

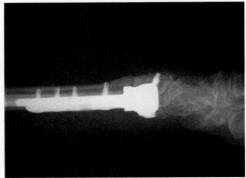

Fig. 13. To assure proper alignment of an ulnar head implant in a patient who has a distal radius malunion, consideration should be given to performing a concurrent corrective osteotomy. (Courtesy of Mayo Clinic College of Medicine, Rochester, MN; with permission.)

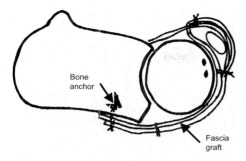

Fig. 14. Schematic of a technique to stabilize an ulnar head implant with soft tissue deficiency using a fascial graft secured to the radius with bone anchors. (Courtesy of Mayo Clinic College of Medicine, Rochester, MN; with permission.)

consider the reconstruction of the dorsal and palmar joint capsules. The authors have used autograft fascia lata and allograft Achilles tendon for this purpose (Fig. 14). Through dorsal and palmar approaches, the strip of fascia/tendon is secured to the dorsal and palmar rims of the sigmoid notch with bone anchors, passing deep to the flexor carpi ulnaris and ECU tendons, and placed under as much tension as possible. The TFCC is secured circumferentially to this band with sutures. The forearm is maintained in neutral rotation for a minimum of 6 weeks post surgery.

Results

Clinical results

van Schoonhoven and colleagues [35] presented promising clinical results with the Martin Ulnar Head prosthesis (Hand Innovations, LLC, Miami, Florida) in a series of 23 patients. This prosthesis, with the articulating head made out of ceramic, is available in three sizes. It is currently not available in the United States. The average follow-up of these investigators' study was 27 months. They showed that remodeling of the sigmoid fossa against the ceramic head of the prosthesis can develop. They reported no signs of prosthetic loosening or primary prosthesis failure.

The authors have experience with the Avanta U-Head prosthesis in 22 patients followed over 2 years. Indications have been primary rheumatoid disease, DRUJ arthritis, and failed distal ulna resections. Soft tissue closure has provided good DRUJ stability in all patients. Clinical results are good to excellent in 18 of the 22 patients (two failures have been successfully revised). In this series, 2 patients required additional soft tissue stabilization during the primary procedure with the Linscheid-Hui ligament reconstruction. The authors found two cases of prosthesis failure (stem loosening). One was related to osteoporosis, requiring revision with a cemented stem, and the

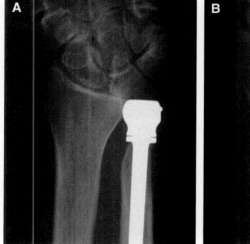
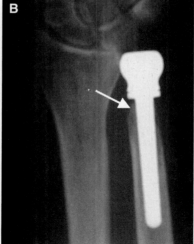

Fig. 15. (A, B) A consistent postoperative finding is radiographic resorption of 2 to 3 mm of distal ulna, just proximal to the implant collar (arrow). This resorption has not resulted in loosening or instability. (Courtesy of Mayo Clinic College of Medicine, Rochester, MN; with permission.)

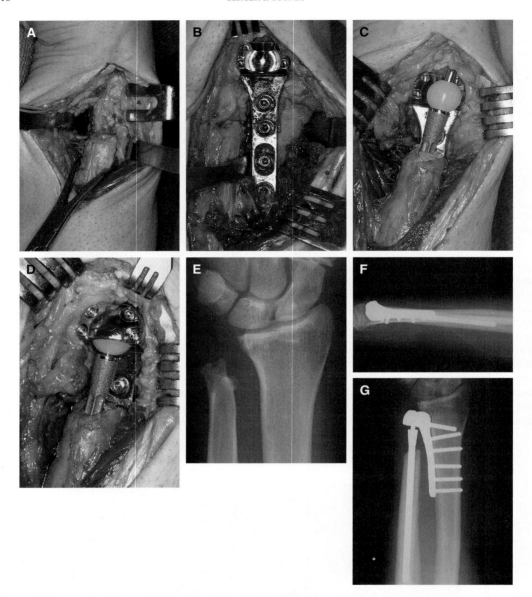

Fig. 16. (*A*) Preparation for an APTIS implant, with the distal end of the ulnar excised, exposing the ulnar cortex of the distal radius metaphysis. (*B*) The radial component of the APTIS implant has been secured to the radius. (*C*) The ulnar stem has been implanted and the polyethylene sphere placed on the stem. (*D*) The cap of the radial component has been placed over the polyethylene sphere. (*E*) Preoperative PA radiograph of a patient who had an unstable forearm following partial excision of the ulna. (*F*) Postoperative lateral radiograph and (*G*) postoperative PA radiograph of the patient illustrated in (*E*) following implantation of the APTIS device. (Courtesy of Mayo Clinic College of Medicine, Rochester, MN; with permission.)

other was in a patient who had a wrist arthrodesis. A third patient required revision secondary to malposition of the ulnar head. A fourth patient has residual dorsal instability but without revision (a fair result). Distal ulnar prosthesis placement

with prior wrist fusion can be difficult for exposure of the ulna shaft. The use of a small burr or awl may be needed, along with careful broaching. An offset broach is made available for cases of previous wrist fusion. All patients demonstrated radiographic resorption of bone just proximal to the collar of the ulnar head implant, which stabilized at an average of 3 mm, 6 months following implantation (Fig. 15). The authors consider this a normal postoperative feature and advise their patients to expect this phenomenon, assuring them that it has not been associated with any problems that they have been able to detect.

Future options

As noted previously, a sigmoid notch hemi-arthroplasty device has been developed but is currently seeking Food and Drug Administration approval. It is anticipated that this device will provide options for dealing with residual instability and bone deficiencies in combination with an ulnar head implant. In addition, the bone-sparing, surface-replacement arthroplasties developed for wrist joint replacement are compatible with the ulnar head implant so long as the sigmoid notch is preserved.

There are limits to how much ulna can be resected and still be compatible with implant arthroplasty. With increasing distances to span, the stem of any implant experiences tremendous strains, especially at the bone–implant interface. Recently, wide resection of the ulna has been advocated as a treatment option for symptomatic failed ulnar head resections. It is unfortunate that excessive ulnar resection has rendered a number of these patients unsuitable for ulnar head hemi-arthroplasty procedures. The authors have had favorable early experience with a newly available device designed by Dr. Luis Scheker (APTIS, Louisville, Kentucky). This implant is a constrained device composed of a curved plate fixed to the radius, a shaft implanted into the medullary canal of the ulna, and a connecting high-density polyethylene sphere contained within a socket integral to the radial plate (Fig. 16). The pistoning of the ulnar component through the polyethylene sphere helps to compensate for the lack of translation. The authors' early results have been encouraging in these difficult situations that have massive resection of distal ulna, but they look forward to longer-term follow-up.

References

[1] Bowers WH. Distal radioulnar joint arthroplasty: the hemiresection—interposition technique. J Hand Surg [Am] 1985;10:169–78.

[2] Darrach W. Partial excision of the lower shaft of the ulna. Ann Surg 1912;56:802–3.

[3] Dingman PVC. Resection of the distal end of the ulna. J Bone Joint Surg Am 1952;34:893–900.

[4] Sotereanos DG, Leit ME. A modified Darrach procedure for treatment of the painful distal radioulnar joint. Clin Orth 1996;325:140–7.

[5] Feldon P, Terrano AL, Belsky MR. Wafer distal ulna resection for triangular fibrocartilage tears and/or ulna impaction syndrome. J Hand Surg Am 1992;17:731–7.

[6] Watson HK, Gabuzda GM. Matched distal ulna resection for posttraumatic disorders of the distal radioulnar joint. J Hand Surg [Am] 1992;17:724–30.

[7] DeSmet LA, Van Ransbeeck H. The Sauve-Kapandji procedure for posttraumatic wrist disorders. Acta Orthop Belg 2000;66:251–4.

[8] Kapandji AI. The Kapandji-Sauvé operation: its techniques and indications in nonrheumatoid diseases. Ann Chir Main 1986;5:181–93.

[9] Lamey DM, Fernandez DL. Results of the modified Sauve-Kapandji procedure in the treatment of chronic posttraumatic derangement of the distal radioulnar joint. J Bone Joint Surg Am 1998;80:1758–69.

[10] Buck-Gramcko D. On the priorities of publication of some operative procedures on the distal end of the ulna. J Hand Surg [Br] 1990;15:416–20.

[11] af Ekenstam F, Engvist O, Wadin K. Results from resection of the distal end of the ulna after fractures of the lower end of the radius. Scand J Plast Reconstr Surg 1982;16:177–81.

[12] Bell MJ, Hill RJ, McMurtry RY. Ulnar impingement syndrome. J Bone Joint Surg Br 1985;67: 126–9.

[13] Bieber EJ, Linscheid RL, Dobyns JH. Failed distal ulna resections. J Hand Surg [Am] 1988;13: 193–200.

[14] Kleinman WB, Greenberg JA. Salvage of the failed Darrach procedure. J Hand Surg [Am] 1995;20: 951–8.

[15] Lees VC, Scheker LR. The radiological demonstration of dynamic ulnar impingement. J Hand Surg [Br] 1997;22:448–50.

[16] McKee MD, Richards RR. Dynamic radio-ulnar convergence after the Darrach procedure. J Bone Joint Surg Br 1996;78:413–8.

[17] Bowers WH. The distal radioulnar joint. In: Green DP, editor. Operative hand surgery. 3rd edition. New York: Churchill Livingstone; 1993. p. 973–1020.

[18] Breen TF, Jupiter JB. Extensor carpi ulnaris and flexor carpi ulnaris tenodesis of the unstable distal ulna. J Hand Sur [Am] 1989;14:612–7.

[19] Gupta R, Allaire RB, Fornalski S, et al. Kinematic analysis of the distal radioulnar joint after a simulated progressive ulnar side wrist injury. J Hand Surg Am 2002;27:854–62.

[20] Hagert CG. Functional aspects of the distal radioulnar joint. J Hand Surg Br 1979;4:585.

[21] Stuart PR, Berger RA, Linscheid RL, et al. The dorsopalmar stability of the distal radioulnar joint. J Hand Surg [Am] 2000;25:689–99.

[22] Blank JE, Cassidy C. The distal radioulnar joint in rheumatoid arthritis. Hand Clin 1996;12:499–513.

[23] Cooney WP, Dobyns WH, Linscheid RL. Complications of Colles' fracture. J Bone Joint Surg Am 1980;62:613–9.

[24] Lichtman DM, Joshi A. Acute injuries of the DRUJ and TFC complex. AAOS Instructional Course Lectures 2003;52:175–83.

[25] Shea K, Fernandez DL, Jupiter JB, et al. Corrective osteotomy for malunited volarly displaced fractures of the distal end of the radius. J Bone Joint Surg Am 1997;79:1816–26.

[26] Stoffelen D, De Smet L, Broos P. The importance of the distal radioulnar joint in distal radius fractures. J Hand Surg [Br] 1998;23:507–11.

[27] Gordon KD, Roth SE, Dunning CE, et al. An arthropometric study of the distal ulna: implications for implant design. J Hand Surg [Am] 2002;27:57–60.

[28] Kapandji IA. The physiology of the joints. Baltimore (MD): Williams & Wilkins; 1979. p. 102–18.

[29] Kapandji AI. Distal radio-ulnar prosthesis. Ann Chir Main 1992;11:320–2.

[30] Kapandi AI. The distal radioulnar joint: functional anatomy. In: Rozemon JP, Fisk GR, editors. The wrist. (GEM Monograph). Edinburgh, UK: Churchill Livingstone; 1988. p. 34.

[31] Masaoka S, Longsworth SH, Werner FW, et al. Biomechanical analyses of two ulnar head prostheses. J Hand Surg [Am] 2002;27:845–53.

[32] Palmer AK, Werner FW. Biomechanics of the distal radioulnar joint. Clin Orthop 1984;187:26–35.

[33] Sauerbier M, Hahn ME, Fujita M, et al. Analysis of dynamic distal radioulnar convergence of the ulna head resection and endoprosthesis implantation. J Hand Surg [Am] 2002;27:425–34.

[34] van Schoonhoven J, Fernandez DL, Bowers WH, et al. Salvage of failed resection arthroplasties of the distal radioulnar joint using a new ulnar head endoprosthesis. J Hand Surg [Am] 2000;25:438–46.

[35] van Schoonhoven J, Herbert TJ, Krimmer H. Neue Konzepte der Endoprothetik des distalen Radioulnargelenkes [A new concept: an endoprosthesis of the distal radioulnar joint]. Handchir Mikrochir Plast Chir 1998;30:387–92.

[36] Sauerbier M, Fujita M, Hahn ME, et al. The dynamic radioulnar convergence of the Darrach procedure and the ulnar head hemi-resection interposition arthroplasty: a biomechanical study. J Hand Surg [Br] 2002;27:307–16.

[37] af Ekenstam F, Hagert CG. Anatomical studies on the geometry and stability of the distal radio ulnar joint. Scand J Plast Reconstr Surg 1985;19:17–25.

[38] DeSmet L, Fabry G. Orientation of the sigmoid notch of the radius: determination of different types of the distal radio-ulnar joint. Acta Orthop Belg 1993;59:269–72.

[39] Berger RA. Arthroscopic anatomy of the wrist and distal radioulnar joint. Hand Clin 1999;15:393–413.

[40] Berger RA. The anatomy of the ligaments of the wrist and distal radioulnar joints. Clin Orthop 2001;383:32–40.

[41] Kauer JMG. The collateral ligament function in the wrist joint. Acta Morphol Neerl Scand 1979;17:252.

[42] Palmer AK, Werner FW. The triangular fibrocartilage complex of the wrist: anatomy and function. J Hand Surg [Am] 1981;6:153–62.

[43] Peterson MS, Adams BD. Biomechanical evaluation of distal radioulnar reconstructions. J Hand Surg [Am] 1993;18:328–34.

[44] Schuind F, An KN, Berglund L, et al. The distal radioulnar joint: a biomechanical study. J Hand Surg [Am] 1991;16:1106–14.

[45] Adams BD, Berger RA. An anatomic reconstruction of the distal radioulnar ligaments for posttraumatic distal radioulnar joint instability. J Hand Surg [Am] 2002;27:243–51.

[46] Haugstvedt JR, Berger RA, Berglund LJ, et al. Development of a dynamic simulator to evaluate distal radio-ulnar joint stability. J Biomech 2001;34:335–9.

[47] Watanabe H, Berger RA, An KN, et al. Stability of the distal radioulnar joint contributed by the joint capsule. J Hand Surg Am 2004;29(6):1114–20.

[48] Viegas SF, Pogue DJ, Patterson RM. Effects of radioulnar instability on the radiocarpal joint. J Hand Surg Am 1990;15:728–32.

[49] Mannerfelt LG. Tendon transfers in surgery of the rheumatoid hand. Hand Clin 1988;4:309–16.

[50] Vaughn-Jackson OJ. Rupture of extensor tendons by attrition of the inferior radioulnar joint. J Bone Joint Surg Br 1948;30:528.

[51] Tsai TM, Schmizu H, Adkins P. A modified extensor carpi ulnaris tenodesis with the Darrach procedure. J Hand Surg [Am] 1993;18:697–702.

[52] Hui FC, Linscheid RL. Lunotriquetral augmentation tenodesis: a reconstruction procedure for dorsal subluxation of the distal radioulnar joint. J Hand Surg [Am] 1982;7:230–6.

[53] Stanley D, Herbert TJ. The Swanson ulnar head prosthesis for post-traumatic disorders of the distal radioulnar joint. J Hand Surg [Br] 1992;17:682–8.

[54] Swanson AB. Implant arthroplasty for disabilities of the distal radioulnar joint: use of a silicone rubber capping implant following resection of the ulnar head. Orthop Clin North Am 1973;4:373–82.

[55] Senachaud C, Savioz D, Della Santa D. Stabilization of the distal radioulnar joint by Hui-Linscheid ligamentoplasty: report of 10 cases. Ann Chir Main Mem Superieur 1996;15:70–9.

ELSEVIER
SAUNDERS

Hand Clin 21 (2005) 621–630

Total Wrist Arthroplasty

Matthew C. Anderson, MD[a], Brian D. Adams, MD[a,b],*

[a]Department of Orthopedic Surgery, University of Iowa, 200 Hawkins Drive, Iowa City, IA 52242, USA
[b]Department of Biomedical Engineering, University of Iowa, 200 Hawkins Drive, Iowa City, IA 52242, USA

Normal wrist motion is accomplished by a complex interaction of multiple articulations involving the radius, ulna, and carpal bones. Total wrist arthroplasty cannot duplicate this intricate system but can potentially produce a stable, pain-free joint with a functional range of motion. A motion-preserving alternative to wrist arthrodesis is of particular importance when treating patients who are debilitated by arthritis that afflicts multiple joints. Total wrist arthroplasty enhances the performance of daily activities and is preferred to arthrodesis by rheumatoid patients [1,2]. Other patients may also choose arthroplasty over arthrodesis to better maintain their ability to perform vocational and avocational activities. Regardless of the need or desire for arthroplasty, the patient must accept and commit to a lifetime of restricted activities imposed by an artificial wrist. The patient must also recognize the risk of implant failure and the consequent need for revision surgery. This article discusses the history, technique, and outcomes of total wrist arthroplasty, with emphasis on new implant designs and strategies to minimize risks and manage complications.

Historical perspective

Swanson [3] designed the first wrist implant to have wide Unites States commercial distribution. The implant is made of silicone that acts as a flexible spacer, and wrist motion results from

a combination of implant flexibility and pistoning within the medullary canals of the radius and metacarpal. Early results were generally gratifying, with good pain relief and an acceptable range of motion; however, restoration of wrist height and hand balance were unpredictable. Longer follow-up revealed subsidence within the bone and a high incidence of implant breakage (Fig. 1), reaching 52% at 72 months [4–6]. Silicone synovitis became an important issue later, although the incidence was lower than with carpal implants [7].

Early articulated total wrist prostheses were semiconstrained and incorporated bearings with small surface areas. These designs were intended to maximize flexion and extension; however, problems with instability and imbalance were common (Fig. 2) [4,8]. Various stem designs for fixation in the radius and carpus were tried. Carpal components were typically fixed in the metacarpal canals with cement. A high incidence of loosening marked by metacarpal erosion and implant penetration occurred. Periprosthetic bone resorption of the distal radius was also common [9]. Early design changes focused on reducing wrist imbalance and distal component loosening by more accurately reproducing normal wrist kinematics through changes in the articulation's position and constraint. The revised Meuli (Sulzer Orthopaedics, Winterthur, Switzerland), Trispherical (Osteonics, Allendale, New Jersey), and revised Voltz (Howmedica, Rutherford, New Jersey) implants each provided satisfactory early clinical results, but further follow-up revealed continued problems with imbalance, subsidence, and loosening [9–15]. The Biax (DePuy, Warsaw, Indiana) prosthesis introduced an ellipsoid-shaped articulation that demonstrated improved wrist balance. Results were good in most patients,

* Corresponding author. University of Iowa, UHIC, Orthopaedics, 200 Hawkins Drive, Iowa City, IA 52242.

E-mail address: brian-d-adams@uiowa.edu (B.D. Adams).

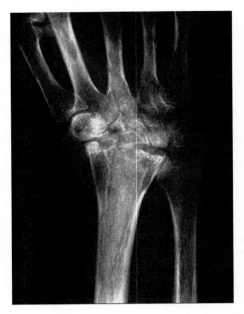

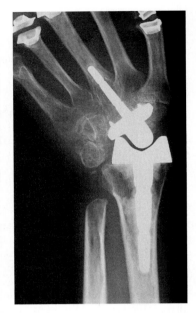

Fig. 1. Swanson silicone wrist implant showing subsidence and breakage at 5 years post surgery.

Fig. 2. Voltz prosthesis showing ulnar deviation imbalance.

but loosening remained a substantial problem. Eight of 11 failures in one series of 58 Biax implants were secondary to distal component loosening and subsidence, which often resulted in penetration through the dorsum of the third metacarpal (Fig. 3). A study investigating the use of the Biax prosthesis incorporating a longer metacarpal stem for primary total wrist arthroplasty in 17 patients who had radiographic evidence of poor bone quality showed more favorable survivorship, with no failures at an average 6-year follow-up [16]. The anatomic physiologic implant (Implant-Service Vertreibs-GmbH, Hamburg, Germany) was designed with a titanium articulation [15]. Midterm follow-up revealed a very high failure rate. Of 40 patients at an average 52-month follow-up, 39 underwent revision to an arthrodesis. Isolated loosening of the carpal component was the most common mode of failure. Titanium wear debris was found in the soft tissues of all revision cases and thought to be the primary contributing factor to early periprosthetic bone resorption [17]. The first-generation Universal prosthesis (Kineticos Medical Incorporated [KMI], Carlsbad, California) combined the concepts of containing fixation within the carpus, augmenting distal component fixation using screws, and performing an intercarpal fusion [18]. The design and method

proved to be more durable, but the bearing shape was prone to instability (Fig. 4).

The overall experience with different designs during the last three and a half decades strongly indicates there are specific criteria to optimize the clinical results [19]. Distal component fixation should primarily be within the carpus rather than relying on the metacarpal canals. It should be combined with a solid intercarpal fusion to provide broad support for the component. Using screws to augment initial fixation has been shown to be effective [20]. The radial component should be shaped to minimize bone resection, which preserves the joint capsule, thereby enhancing prosthetic stability and wrist balance. In patients who have adequate bone quality, fixation by osteointegration rather than cement would seem to be a better choice for both components to improve durability and reduce bone destruction if revision is necessary. The articulation should be broad, generally ellipsoidal in shape, and semiconstrained [19]. It should also resist imbalance and instability yet provide a functional range of motion that can be achieved early with minimal formal rehabilitation. Finally, there should be the option to preserve the ulnar head and distal radioulnar joint (DRUJ). These criteria were incorporated in the design of the Universal 2 implant (Kineticos Medical Incorporated [KMI],

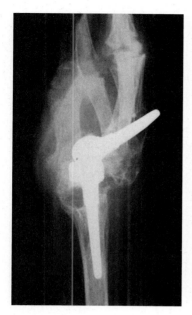

Fig. 3. Biax prosthesis with distal component migration and penetration through the dorsum of the third metacarpal.

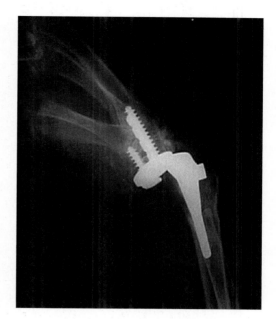

Fig. 4. Universal 2 prosthesis with volar dislocation of the carpal component.

San Diego, California) (Fig. 5) and other implants that are under development.

Patient selection

The objective of total wrist arthroplasty is to maintain or improve wrist motion while relieving pain and correcting deformity. Patients who have the greatest need for maintaining wrist motion are those afflicted by arthritis involving multiple upper-extremity joints and those who have specific needs or desires to maintain motion. Patients who have rheumatoid arthritis and have bilateral wrist arthritis and elbow and shoulder involvement are particularly good candidates. Individuals who have had a wrist fusion on one side and total wrist arthroplasty on the other prefer arthroplasty [2,9]. Basic activities of daily living such as perineal care, fastening buttons, combing hair, and writing are made easier if some wrist motion, particularly flexion, is preserved [21,22]. Patients who have post-traumatic or degenerative osteoarthritis may also be proper candidates for total wrist arthroplasty. Because these patients typically have good bone quality, muscle strength, and wrist alignment, the result can be excellent. This type of patient, however, should choose arthroplasty to maintain dexterity for activities of daily living and specific low-demand activities rather than to increase activity levels and must be willing to accept permanent activity restrictions.

In patient selection, it is perhaps more important to consider contraindications rather than indications. Most patients with post-traumatic arthritis are young and very active and, thus, are not candidates for arthroplasty due to the high stresses imposed on the wrist. Likewise, some patients with osteoarthritis plan to remain active in physically demanding activities for many years. Rheumatoid patients with highly active synovitis that is producing severe bony erosions or joint hyperlaxity have a higher risk for implant instability and loosening. These patients are better treated by arthrodesis. Regular use of the upper extremities for support during ambulation or transfers is a contraindication; however, intermittent use of crutches or a cane is acceptable if the patient uses a wrist splint. Absolute contraindications for total wrist arthroplasty include a minimally functional hand, recent infection, and lack of wrist extension power due to ruptures of the extensor carpi radialis brevis and longus tendons or a radial nerve palsy.

There must be adequate bone stock and quality to support the implant, especially the carpal component. Implantation in patients who have

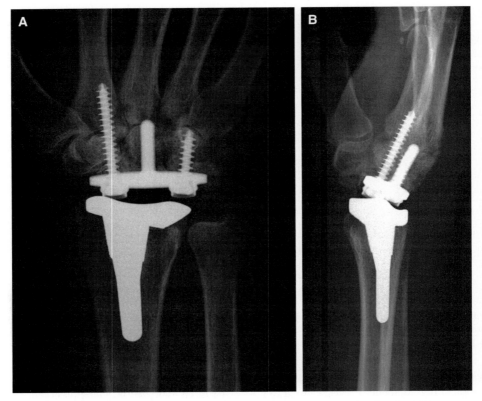

Fig. 5. (*A, B*) Universal 2 implant, with preservation of the ulnar head and DRUJ.

severe ostoeopenia, bone erosion, or joint deformity is more challenging, and the implant fixation is less durable. Previous surgical fusion or proximal row carpectomy are relative contraindications. These patients must have adequate carpus remaining and intact wrist extensors to convert to an arthroplasty. Although the procedure is more technically challenging after these procedures, the implantation and functional outcome can be very good.

Preoperative planning

Patients with rheumatoid arthritis should have a full preoperative evaluation including the cervical spine. Total hip or knee replacement should be performed before wrist arthroplasty to avoid weight bearing on the wrist prosthesis during rehabilitation. Wrist replacement may be done before or after shoulder or elbow surgery but should usually be performed before procedures on the digits to optimize joint alignment and tendon tension in the hand. To reduce the risk of infection and wound healing problems, temporarily stopping medications such as methotrexate and other immune-modulating medications should be considered after consulting with the patient's rheumatologist. The risk of bleeding complications is reduced by decreasing or eliminating nonsteroidal anti-inflammatory drugs for at least 10 days before and 5 days after surgery.

Radiographic assessment of bone quality, erosions, carpal collapse, carpal ulnar translation, volar subluxation, and the condition of the DRUJ prepares the surgeon to optimize the technique and avoid potential difficulties. Implant size and alignment within the bones can be predicted using radiographic templates.

Operative technique

Although the technique for implantation of the Universal 2 (Kineticos Medical Incorporated [KMI], San Diego, California) is described in this article, it has many similarities to other systems currently in use.

Templating

In the posteroanterior (PA) view, the radial component should not extend beyond the edge of the radial styloid. The carpal component should not extend more than 2 mm over the margins of the carpus at the level of the osteotomy. In general, the smaller implant should be selected when deciding between two sizes. The optimum size is typically found when the carpal stem is aligned with the center of capitate and the ulnar screw enters the proximal pole of the hamate.

Exposure

Preoperative antibiotic is administered. An arm tourniquet is used. A wide strip of adhesive drape is applied to the dorsum of the wrist and hand to help protect the skin. A dorsal longitudinal incision is made over the wrist in line with the third metacarpal. The skin and the subcutaneous tissue are elevated together to reduce the risk of skin necrosis and to protect the sensory branches of the radial and ulnar nerves. The sixth dorsal extensor compartment is opened along its volar margin. The entire retinaculum is elevated radially to the septum between the first and second extensor compartments. An extensor tenosynovectomy is performed if needed. The integrity of the extensor carpi radialis brevis and longus are confirmed.

The dorsal wrist capsule is raised in continuity with the dorsal DRUJ capsule and the periosteum over the distal 1 cm of the radius as a distally based rectangular flap (Fig. 6). If the distal ulna is to be preserved, then the interval between the capsule and the dorsal distal radioulnar ligament is carefully divided and the capsule is raised distally to preserve the horizontal components of the triangular fibrocartilage complex. The sides of the flap are made in the floors of the first and sixth extensor compartments. The brachioradialis and first extensor compartment are elevated subperiosteally from the distal portion of the radial styloid. The wrist is fully flexed to expose the joint. Synovectomies of the radiocarpal joint and DRUJ are performed when needed. If the DRUJ is arthritic, then the distal ulna is resected through its neck or rounded to create a hemiresection arthroplasty of the DRUJ.

Radial component

Preparation for radial component implantation begins by inserting an alignment rod into the

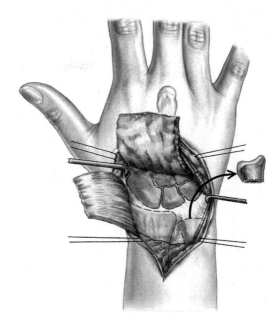

Fig. 6. Exposure of the distal radius and carpus using a radially based retinacular flap and distally based capsular flap. Ulnar head excision is optional.

canal of the radius. To insert the rod, a hole is made with an awl about 5 mm volar to the dorsal lip of the distal radius, just radial to Lister's tubercle. Fluoroscopy confirms central placement of the rod in the canal (Fig. 7). The radial guide bar and cutting block are mounted on the rod and positioned to remove only the articular surface. Lister's tubercle may need to be removed for full seating of the block. After temporary fixation pins are inserted through the block, the alignment rod is removed, and the osteotomy is performed with an oscillating saw (Fig. 8). If the DRUJ is to be preserved, then the cut is stopped approximately 5 mm short of the sigmoid notch; the jig is removed and the cut is completed with the saw by free-hand technique, whereby it flares slightly ulnarward and out through the distal articular surface of the radius. The cutting block and pins are removed, the guide rod is reinserted, and the appropriate-sized intramedullary broach is mounted on the rod. The broach is aligned with the sigmoid notch and dorsal rim of the radius and driven into the radius until its collar becomes flush with the cortex. (Fig. 9). A trial radial component is inserted. The carpus can be reduced on the radial component to assess soft tissue tension. If it is excessive, then further resection of the

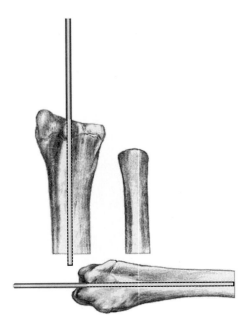

Fig. 7. A guide rod inserted to align cutting block and broach for radius preparation.

radius may be necessary but is usually delayed until the carpal preparation is completed.

In preparing the carpus, the scaphoid and triquetrum are temporarily pinned (if they are mobile) to facilitate the osteotomy. The lunate is

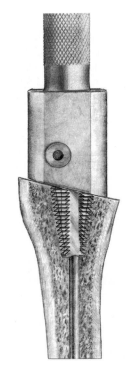

Fig. 9. Radius is broached using a cannulated broach over a guide rod.

excised by sharp dissection or rongeur. Using the drill guide, a hole is made in the center of the capitate. The carpal guide bar is inserted in the hole. The carpal cutting block is applied and positioned to resect the proximal 1 mm of hamate, a small amount of the capitate head, and about half of the scaphoid and triquetrum (Fig. 10). The cutting block is held with temporary fixation pins. The osteotomy is made with a small oscillating saw.

The trial carpal component is inserted, and the holes for the screws are made using the drill guide. The radial drill hole passes through the scaphoid, trapezium, and second carpometacarpal (CMC) joint to a depth of 30 to 35 mm (Fig. 11). The hole is typically not perpendicular to the carpal component, but the screws and the component are designed to accommodate oblique screw angles. Again, using the drill guide, the ulnar hole is made into the hamate to a depth of 15 to 20 mm but does not cross the mobile CMC joint.

The trial screws for the carpal component are inserted and the trial poly component is applied. The prosthesis is reduced and its motion and stability are tested. It is typically quite stable and

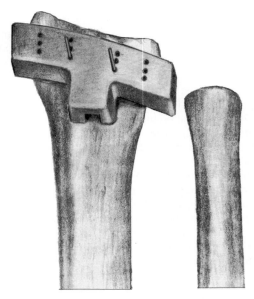

Fig. 8. Radial cutting block is applied to resect the articular surface at the proper angle.

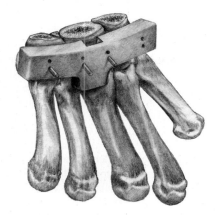

Fig. 10. A carpal cutting block is applied to guide the osteotomy through the capitate head, scaphoid waist, and midtriquetrum.

should demonstrate approximately 35° of flexion and 35° of extension, with modest tightness at full extension. If the volar capsule is limiting extension, then the radius may need to be shortened slightly (2 mm). When a preoperative flexion contracture is present, a step-cut tendon lengthening of the wrist flexors may be necessary. Conversely, when tension is insufficient, the palmar joint capsule is inspected and repaired when

detached. If the capsule is intact, however, a thicker polyethylene may be required.

Before implanting the final prosthesis, three horizontal mattress sutures of 2-0 polyester are placed through small bone holes along the dorsal rim of the distal radius for eventual capsule closure. If the ulnar head was resected, then sutures are also placed through the dorsal neck. The articular surfaces are removed from the triquetrum, capitate, hamate, scaphoid, and trapezoid and previously resected bone is packed into the spaces to achieve an intercarpal arthrodesis. The final implants are impacted into place and the final screws are inserted tightly. The capsule should be repaired to completely enclose the implants. The extensor retinaculum is repaired, leaving the extensor carpi radialis longus and brevis and the extensor pollicis longus superficial to the retinaculum. The skin is closed over a self-suction drain, and a volar plaster wrist splint is applied.

Postoperative management

The postoperative dressing and plaster splint are removed on day 2 and a supervised exercise program is begun, including full digital motion

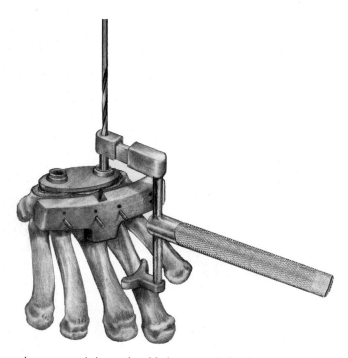

Fig. 11. Trial carpal component is inserted and holes are made for the screws using a special drill guide.

and gentle active wrist motion (flexion, extension, radial and ulnar deviation, pronation, supination). Wrist extension is specifically emphasized. Strengthening is added at week 4, and full activities permitted after 8 weeks. The patient is advised to avoid impact loading of the wrist (eg, use of a hammer, playing tennis) and repetitive forceful use of the hand. In general, patients are advised to only intermittently lift greater than 10 lb.

Results

In Menon's [18] first report of 37 Universal 2 prostheses with a mean follow-up of 6.7 years (range, 4–10 years), no case demonstrated radiographic evidence of distal component loosening. In a further follow-up study that included 57 implants, carpal component loosening was again not reported [23]. Subsidence of the radial component was observed but was not progressive or symptomatic. Similar to other prostheses, the Universal 2 implant provided consistently good pain relief (90%) and a functional range of motion. Average postoperative motion was 36° extension, 41° flexion, 7° radial deviation, and 13° ulnar deviation. Dislocation was the most common complication, with five occurring in the first 37 cases and six among the 57 cases in the later follow-up.

A prospective study of 22 Universal 2 prosthesis implanted by two surgeons with a 1- to 2-year follow-up demonstrated results similar to Menon's [18]. Patients achieved an average of 41° flexion and 35° extension [20]. Disabilities of the Arm, Shoulder, and Hand (DASH) outcome survey scores improved 24 points at 2 years. Three prostheses (14%) were unstable and required further treatment; these were in patients with highly active rheumatoid disease with severe wrist laxity. A further multicenter study of 53 patients again showed good results at 1- to 5-year follow-up, with nearly equivalent outcomes of motion and patient satisfaction achieved by all surgeons [24]. Dislocation continued to occur, with a 9% overall incidence. Distal component loosening occurred in 4 patients, of whom all had persistently active synovitis and failed to achieve an intercarpal fusion, resulting in lack of solid bony implant support.

In addition to the results previously described, a midterm follow-up of 66 Biax wrists showed good pain relief and good subjective outcome at a mean of 52 months post surgery. Five of the replacements were revised or fused because of loosening, and an additional 9 showed radiographic signs of loosening [25]. Another short-term study of 16 Biax wrists showed good-to-excellent results in 69% at a mean 25-month follow-up. Four early dislocations occurred, one of which was revised [26]. Although the Biax wrist implant provided satisfactory results in many patients, it is no longer commercially available.

The Avanta total wrist (Avanta Orthopedics, San Diego, California) was introduced approximately 2 years ago. It offers a mobile bearing attached to the carpal component that theoretically improves load transfer and reduces stresses that could cause loosening. Similar to the first-generation Universal prosthesis, the proximal and distal components are cemented. There have been no published reports on the outcome of this prosthesis.

Early results with the Universal 2 prosthesis in 25 patients (20 women and 5 men) operated by two surgeons have been excellent. Twenty patients had rheumatoid arthritis, 2 had post-traumatic arthritis, and 3 had osteoarthritis. All prostheses were implanted uncemented. Results revealed excellent fixation, with an average of 37° flexion, 33° extension, 22° ulnar deviation, and 9° radial deviation. Pain relief was rated good by all patients but mild ulnar-sided wrist discomfort persisted in 5. Pain relief and motion often did not reach their maximum improvements for 6 months. Average DASH scores improved 20% and patient rated wrist evaluation scores improved 35%. No cases showed radiographic implant loosening, but 1 osteopenic patient had 3 mm of subsidence that plateaued. There have been no dislocations and no implant loosenings or revisions [27]. An additional surgeon survey found no reported dislocations or revisions in over 125 wrists implanted in the United States.

In the initial group of 20 patients, the carpal component stem fractured between the first and second postoperative year in 3 patients who had the first version of this implant. The carpal component was subsequently redesigned to have a greater diameter, a stronger stem, and a full porous coating over its entire distal surface (stem and plate) for better durability and osteointegration. No fractures have been found with the revised version of the carpal component.

Potential complications

Potential intraoperative complications include fractures and tendon injury, which can be treated at that time. Possible postoperative complications include wound healing problems (hematoma, wound edge necrosis, dehiscence), extensor tendon adhesions, wrist stiffness, wrist imbalance, DRUJ problems (impingement, instability, arthrosis), prosthetic instability, aseptic loosening, and infection. The true incidence of these complications for the newest designs of wrist replacement currently in use is unknown but appears to be low during the first 2 postoperative years. With the exceptions of advanced loosening and infection, each of these complications is treated based on the perspective of the patient's needs and desires.

Failed total wrist arthroplasty

Revision arthroplasty, arthrodesis, and resection arthroplasty are options for salvaging a failed total wrist arthroplasty due to imbalance, loosening, or instability. Revision arthroplasty is an option for aseptic loosening if there is adequate bone stock or if bone grafting is feasible. The thickened capsule must be widely released to allow wrist flexion and extraction of the components. If there has been substantial subsidence, then lengthening of the wrist flexors and extensor tendons may be required. Iliac crest bone graft may be needed to fill defects and re-establish the basic architecture of the carpus. When using the Universal 2 prosthesis for revision, the graft can be transfixed to the remaining carpus using the carpal component fixation screws. Because the decision to perform a revision depends primarily on the integrity of the bone and soft tissues, it may not be possible to decide until direct inspection at the time of surgery. Thus, the surgeon must be prepared for arthroplasty and for arthrodesis. Patients who have poor bone stock, severe capsule defects, or particulate synovitis are rarely indicated for revision arthroplasty. An established infection should be treated by implant removal and by primary or delayed conversion to an arthrodesis [8,28,29].

Summary

Total wrist arthroplasty preserves motion and improves hand function for daily tasks and lower-demand vocational and avocational activities. It is often preferable to fusion when both wrists are arthritic. Newer prosthetic designs provide a functional range of motion, better wrist balance, reduced risk of loosening, and better implant stability than older designs. The success of total wrist arthroplasty depends on appropriate patient selection, careful preoperative planning, and sound surgical technique.

References

[1] Goodman MJ, Millender LH, Nalebuff ED, et al. Arthroplasty of the rheumatoid wrist with silicone rubber: an early evaluation. J Hand Surg [Am] 1980;5(2):114–21.

[2] Vicar AJ, Burton RI. Surgical management of the rheumatoid wrist—fusion or arthroplasty. J Hand Surg [Am] 1986;11(6):790–7.

[3] Swanson AB. Flexible implant arthroplasty for arthritic disabilities of the radiocarpal joint. A silicone rubber intramedullary stemmed flexible hinge implant for the wrist joint. Orthop Clin North Am 1973;4(2):383–94.

[4] Jolly SL, Ferlic DC, Clayton ML, et al. Swanson silicone arthroplasty of the wrist in rheumatoid arthritis: a long-term follow-up. J Hand Surg [Am] 1992; 17(1):142–9.

[5] Fatti JF, Palmer AK, Mosher JF. The long-term results of Swanson silicone rubber interpositional wrist arthroplasty. J Hand Surg [Am] 1986;11(2): 166–75.

[6] Stanley JK, Tolat AR. Long-term results of Swanson Silastic arthroplasty in the rheumatoid wrist. J Hand Surg [Br] 1993;18(3):381–8.

[7] Peimer CA, Medige J, Eckert BS, et al. Reactive synovitis after silicone arthroplasty. J Hand Surg [Am] 1986;11(5):624–38.

[8] Ferlic DC, Jolly SN, Clayton ML. Salvage for failed implant arthroplasty of the wrist. J Hand Surg [Am] 1992;17(5):917–23.

[9] Meuli H. Total wrist arthroplasty. Experience with a noncemented wrist prosthesis. Clin Orthop 1997; 342:77–83.

[10] Dennis DA, Ferlic DC, Clayton ML. Volz total wrist arthroplasty in rheumatoid arthritis: a long-term review. J Hand Surg [Am] 1986;11(4):483–90.

[11] Menon J. Total wrist replacement using the modified Volz prosthesis. J Bone Joint Surg Am 1987;69(7): 998–1006.

[12] Figgie MP, Inglis AE, Sobel M, et al. Trispherical total wrist arthroplasty in rheumatoid arthritis. J Hand Surg [Am] 1990;15(2):217–23.

[13] Cobb TK, Beckenbaugh RD. Biaxial total-wrist arthroplasty. J Hand Surg [Am] 1996;21(6):1011–21.

[14] Cobb TK, Beckenbaugh RD. Biaxial long-stemmed multipronged distal components for revision/bone deficit total-wrist arthroplasty. J Hand Surg [Am] 1996;21(5):764–70.

[15] Radmer S, Andresen R, Sparmann M. Wrist arthroplasty with a new generation of prostheses in patients with rheumatoid arthritis. J Hand Surg [Am] 1999;24(5):935–43.

[16] Rizzo M, Beckenbaugh RD. Results of biaxial total wrist arthroplasty with a modified (long) metacarpal stem. J Hand Surg [Am] 2003;28(4):577–84.

[17] Radmer S, Andresen R, Sparmann M. Total wrist arthroplasty in patients with rheumatoid arthritis. J Hand Surg [Am] 2003;28(5):789–94.

[18] Menon J. Universal Total Wrist Implant: experience with a carpal component fixed with three screws. J Arthroplasty 1998;13(5):515–23.

[19] Grosland NM, Rogge RD, Adams BD. Influence of articular geometry on prosthetic wrist stability. Clin Orthop 2004;412:134–42.

[20] Divelbiss BJ, Sollerman C, Adams BD. Early results of the Universal total wrist arthroplasty in rheumatoid arthritis. J Hand Surg [Am] 2002; 27(2):195–204.

[21] Hastings H. Total wrist arthrodesis for post traumatic conditions. Indiana Hand Cent Newslett 1994;1:14–8.

[22] Millender LH, Nalebuff EA. Arthrodesis of the rheumatoid wrist. An evaluation of sixty patients and a description of a different surgical technique. J Bone Joint Surg Am 1973;55(5):1026–34.

[23] Menon J. Total wrist arthroplasty for rheumatoid arthritis. In: Saffar P, Goucher G, editors. Current practice in hand surgery. London: Martin Dunitz; 1997. p. 209–14.

[24] Adams BD. A multicenter study of the Universal Total Wrist Prosthesis. Presented at the 57th Annual Meeting of the American Society for Surgery of the Hand. Phoenix, Arizona, 2002.

[25] Takwale VJ, Nuttall D, Trail IA, et al. Biaxial total wrist replacement in patients with rheumatoid arthritis. J Bone Joint Surg Br 2002;84:692–9.

[26] Stegeman M, Rijnberg WJ, van Loon CJM. Biaxial total wrist arthroplasty in rheumatoid arthritis. Rheumatol Int 2005;25:191–4.

[27] Adams BD. Universal 2 Total Wrist Arthroplasty. Presented at the 55th Annual Meeting of the Association of Bone and Joint Surgeons. Paris, 2003.

[28] Lorei MP, Figgie MP, Ranawat CS, et al. Failed total wrist arthroplasty. Analysis of failures and results of operative management. Clin Orthop 1997;342:84–93.

[29] Cooney WP III, Beckenbaugh RD, Linscheid RL. Total wrist arthroplasty. Problems with implant failures. Clin Orthop 1984;187:121–8.

Wrist Arthrodesis

Radford J. Hayden, PA-C[a,b], Peter J.L. Jebson, MD[a,*]

[a]*Division of Elbow, Hand, and Microsurgery, Department of Orthopaedic Surgery,*
University of Michigan Health Systems, 2098 South Main Street, Ann Arbor, MI 48103, USA
[b]*College of Health Professions, Physician Assistant Studies,*
University of Detroit Mercy, P.O. Box 19900, Detroit, MI 48219-0900, USA

Complete or total wrist arthrodesis is a well established reconstructive surgical procedure that results in predictable pain relief and satisfactory function in patients who have various inflammatory, degenerative, and post-traumatic conditions. First described in the early 1900s, the goal of wrist arthrodesis is to provide the patient with a stable wrist for power grip and the predictable relief of pain while sacrificing wrist motion. Numerous techniques and fixation devices have been described to achieve a successful fusion of the radius to the carpus. The most popular techniques involve intramedullary rod or dorsal plate and screw fixation in conjunction with autogenous cancellous bone graft from the iliac crest or distal radius. Despite the loss of wrist motion, most patients report satisfactory functional outcomes, confirming that they are able to accomplish most daily activities of living with some adaptation and compensation. Wrist arthrodesis is an acceptable treatment approach for those patients in whom a limited arthrodesis or total wrist arthroplasty is contraindicated.

History of wrist arthrodesis

The first reported case of a wrist arthrodesis was by Ely in 1910, who performed the fusion between the base of the third metacarpal and the distal radius using an anterior tibial graft that was sutured into place. The procedure was performed in patients who had wrists afflicted with

tuberculosis [1,2]. Steindler used the complete wrist arthrodesis for the treatment of a patient who had a "drop hand" secondary to a post-traumatic nerve injury following a humerus fracture [3]. He also recommended the procedure for those patients who had a deformed wrist secondary to polio or spastic paresis. In 1923, Gil introduced the concept of the turnabout radial graft in which a 2–3-inch corticocancellous segment of the dorsal distal radius is excised and rotated 180° in the coronal plane before being placed into a denuded tissue bed that included a small cleft in the capitate [4]. In 1942, Abbot and colleagues published the results of their experience with the use of an iliac crest cancellous bone graft for wrist arthrodesis [5]. Colonna in 1944 described the use of a rib graft split longitudinally with the medial portion placed over the dorsum of the wrist and into the second and third metacarpal bases [6]. Wickstrom modified the rib graft technique by inserting the proximal portion of the donor graft into the medullary canal of the distal radius and deepening the cleft at the bases of the second and third metacarpals [7]. Wedge arthrodesis was described by Evans in 1955, in which the distal radius was shaped into a wedge before being inserted into the carpus combined with resection of the lower end of the ulna [8].

With the advent of metallic fixation devices, newer and reportedly simpler methods for achieving a predictable wrist fusion were developed. In 1964, Campbell and Keokarn described an inlay technique to achieve a fusion in the patient who had Kienbock's disease [9]. The lunate was excised, as was the surrounding diseased soft tissue, and an autogenous iliac crest bone graft was shaped to fit the deformity followed by fixation with Kirschner

* Corresponding author.

E-mail address: pjebson@med.umich.edu (P.J.L. Jebson).

wires. Haddad and Riordan proposed an alternative radial approach to the wrist with iliac crest bone graft and K-wire fixation [10]. They advocated such an approach to preserve forearm pronation and supination and to avoid adhesions of the extensor tendons. In 1965, Clayton and others described the use of a large Steinmann pin to fuse the rheumatoid wrist (Fig. 1) [11]. In 1971, Mannerfelt and Malmsten modified the procedure by using a Rush rod inserted through the third metacarpal into the shaft of the radius in conjunction with a Wiberg staple to secure rotational stability [12]. In 1974, Larsson reported a series of 23 cases of successful wrist arthrodesis using a dorsal compression plate from the distal radius across the carpus to the base of the second metacarpal [13]. Dorsal plate fixation has remained popular in patients who have degenerative or post-traumatic arthritis (Fig. 2). Bracey, McMurtry, and Walton used a T-plate between the second and third metacarpals and the distal radius to position the wrist in slight dorsiflexion and ulnar deviation [14]. Wright and McMurtry subsequently reported a large series of 83 patients who underwent an arthrodesis of the wrist with dorsal plate fixation with an overall fusion rate of 96% [15].

Various other modifications of the surgical technique have been described. Benkeddach and colleagues used multiple staples to achieve a stable arthrodesis in the nonrheumatoid patient [16]. Louis and colleagues described a modified proximal row carpectomy and a subsequent radius to capitate arthrodesis with K-wire fixation in patients who had a severely contracted wrist [17]. Wood described a modification of the Gil technique using a combination of Kirschner and tension band wiring [18] (Fig. 3), and Tannenbaum and Louis further modified the technique by using 3.5-mm cortical screws (Fig. 4) [19].

More recently described methods of fixation have included the use of a bioabsorbable poly-l-lactide (POLA) rod as reported by Voutilainen and colleagues [20] and the use of a custom designed precontoured plate with the purported advantages of avoiding prolonged cast immobilization and extensor tendon complications [21,22].

Indications and contraindications for wrist arthrodesis

The most common indication for a complete wrist arthrodesis is the active individual who suffers from degenerative, inflammatory, postinfectious, or post-traumatic radiocarpal and midcarpal arthritis and who remains symptomatic

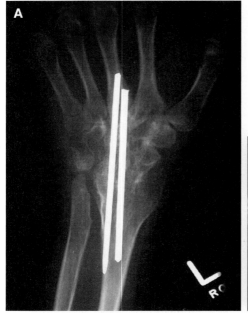
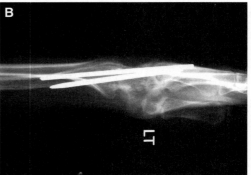

Fig. 1. Wrist arthrodesis using two Steinmann pins.

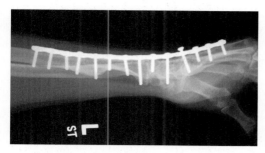

Fig. 2. Dorsal plate and screw fixation was used for the arthrodesis in a patient who had post-traumatic arthritis of the wrist. Note how the plate has been contoured to achieve slight wrist dorsiflexion.

despite the exhaustive use of nonoperative treatment modalities [23]. Additional indications include those conditions that result in instability, destruction, or contracture of the wrist, such as a failed implant arthroplasty or limited intercarpal arthrodesis, a severe flexion deformity of the wrist secondary to spasticity, or bone loss following trauma or tumor resection [23,24].

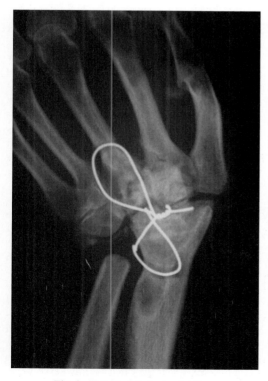

Fig. 3. Tension band wire fixation.

Absolute contraindications for total wrist arthrodesis do exist and include the presence of an open distal radius epiphyseal plate in the skeletally immature patient, the absence of satisfactory soft tissue coverage, and the presence of an active wrist infection. Arthrodesis is also contraindicated in the elderly, sedentary individual who would be better served by a total wrist arthroplasty and the preservation of motion, in the tetraplegic patient who uses their hands in a modified form for grasping and transfer activities, and in those patients for whom a motion-preserving procedure is feasible.

Controversy continues to exist regarding the role of bilateral wrist arthrodeses. In general, those patients who have bilateral wrist disease seem to have a satisfactory outcome when one wrist is fused and the other undergoes implant arthroplasty. Arthrodesis of the nondominant extremity combined with implant arthroplasty of the dominant extremity has been advocated [23]. A consensus regarding the ideal position of the fusion in the patient who requires bilateral wrist arthrodeses does not exist. Brumfield and Champoux recommended 10° of extension for both extremities [25], whereas Rayan and colleagues recommended 5°–10° of flexion for the nondominant wrist and the neutral position for the dominant wrist [26]. Clayton and Ferlic recommended the neutral position for both wrists [27].

Indications and surgical techniques for patients who have inflammatory arthritis

Of the myriad of inflammatory arthritides, rheumatoid arthritis (RA) represents the most common cause of wrist joint destruction necessitating surgical treatment. Several operative procedures exist for the treatment of the rheumatoid wrist with early intervention directed primarily at synovectomy and soft tissue reconstruction. Complete wrist arthrodesis is the most common bony procedure performed in the rheumatoid wrist [28]. The indications for surgical intervention are not based on the radiographic appearance of the wrist per se, because many severely deformed joints are surprisingly minimally painful and the patient's functional abilities remain satisfactory. The patient's age, pain level, functional demands, and their response to previous soft tissue procedures dictate the need for and timing of wrist arthrodesis. The severity of bilateral wrist disease and the presence of rheumatoid changes in the small joints

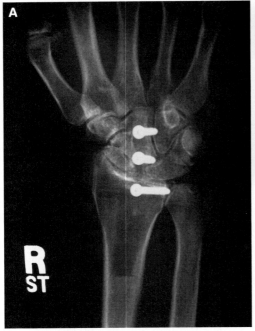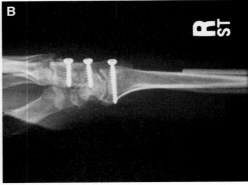

Fig. 4. Wrist arthrodesis accomplished with a turnabout graft stabilized with screws. (Courtesy of Dean S. Louis, MD, Ann Arbor, MI.)

of the hand, elbow, and shoulder are additional considerations [29].

The indications for arthrodesis of the rheumatoid wrist include a destroyed, unstable, painful, and weak wrist that may be also accompanied by ankylosis with flexion or a flexion deformity secondary to rupture of the wrist extensor tendons (ECRL, ECRB) [11,30]. Arthrodesis of the rheumatoid wrist in a position of function also may result in improved motion and function of the digits of the involved hand [30,31]. Finally, complete arthrodesis is a useful salvage procedure following a failed implant arthroplasty [32–34].

Wrist arthrodesis has been accomplished using autogenous cancellous or corticocancellous bone graft from the distal radius or iliac crest. Surgeons have advocated stabilization of the fusion site with K-wire fixation or intramedullary Steinmann pins or Rush rods [12,35–37]. Mohty and Shapiro proposed a two-pin technique with one intramedullary rod placed through the metacarpal of the index finger into the radius and another from the fourth metacarpal into the ulna combined with an ulnar ostectomy [38]. Masada and colleagues described the use of K-wires driven through the second and fourth metacarpal bases

into the distal radius accompanied by autogenous iliac crest bone graft [39].

The use of a dorsal plate and screw fixation for a wrist arthrodesis has been described in the patient who has rheumatoid arthritis, but concerns have been raised about the quality of the bone and the risk for failure of fixation [27]. Regardless of the type of fixation used, arthrodesis of the rheumatoid wrist usually is accompanied by an extensive synovectomy and excision of the ulnar head or arthrodesis of the distal radioulnar joint (DRUJ).

The exact position of the arthrodesis is determined individually and is influenced by the functional and avocational needs of the patient and the status of the opposite wrist. In general, 10°–15° of dorsiflexion and slight ulnar deviation is desirable, although patients experience satisfactory function with the dominant hand fused in the neutral position [35,38,40]. It has been suggested that in patients who have bilateral wrist arthrodeses, the dominant hand be placed in the neutral position and the nondominant hand be placed in some degree of palmar flexion to assist in activities of daily activity that require a slightly flexed wrist, such as perineal care.

Indications and surgical techniques for patients who have degenerative or post-traumatic arthritis

Advanced degenerative arthritis of the wrist involving the radiocarpal and midcarpal articulations, such as that encountered in the scapholunate advanced collapse pattern of wrist arthritis (SLAC wrist), is a well recognized indication for wrist arthrodesis. Another common indication is the presence of post-traumatic arthritis following a complex fracture or fracture–dislocation involving the distal radius or carpus or avascular necrosis of the carpus [41]. Malunion of a severely comminuted intra-articular fracture of the distal radius, or the scaphoid nonunion advanced collapse (SNAC) deformity are other common causes of advanced degeneration necessitating surgical treatment. In recent years, treatment has been directed toward motion sparing procedures, if feasible, with variable success [41,42]. Occasionally the extent of degeneration is limited, permitting such procedures. If they fail, however, a complete arthrodesis usually is indicated [42].

Unlike the numerous surgical techniques described for achieving an arthrodesis in the patient who has inflammatory arthritis, the gold standard for the patient who has post-traumatic or degenerative arthritis is dorsal plate and screw fixation. There are several fixation devices from which to choose, including a low-contact plating system that was developed specifically to reduce the incidence of extensor tendon irritation postoperatively. Titanium or stainless steel implant systems are available. Straight or precontoured plates are also available. The precontoured feature was conceived because of the difficulties encountered with precise contouring of the plate to achieve slight wrist extension and ulnar deviation. Regardless of the plating system selected, the plate typically is fixed to the distal radius, carpus, and third metacarpal. The second metacarpal shaft can be used if necessary and has been advocated to improve positioning of the hand in ulnar deviation. The fusion site usually is supplemented with autologous cancellous bone graft harvested from the distal radius metaphysis or from the iliac crest in those patients who have poor bone quality or a large defect [42–45]. The radioscaphoid, radiolunate, scapholunate, scaphocapitate, and lunocapitate articulations routinely are incorporated into the fusion mass. Controversy exists with respect to the need to incorporate the third carpometacarpal (CMC) articulation. Proponents of including the third CMC joint in the fusion mass maintain

that symptomatic motion is common postoperatively. Variations of the dorsal plate technique also have been reported with variable success for the salvage of a failed total wrist arthroplasty [33,34].

Indications and surgical techniques for the pediatric patient and those who have an unstable or contracted wrist

Those children who require a complete wrist arthrodesis typically present with a flail wrist secondary to a severe birth trauma-related brachial plexus injury or acquired following trauma, or with a severe flexion contracture associated with cerebral palsy, arthrogryposis, or fibrodysplasia ossificans progressiva [46].

One of the earliest cases of a wrist arthrodesis in children was by Epstein, who described an arthrodesis performed by Steindler on a child with infantile paralysis [47]. Nissen noted that a severe flexion contracture of the hand is cosmetically and functionally unacceptable in children and recommended simple tenotomy of the main flexors of the wrist accompanied by Brockman's "gouge" arthrodesis of the wrist [48].

Typically children who have a spastic flexion contracture of the wrist caused by cerebral palsy or arthrogryposis have several clinical factors that influence surgical decision making, including the type of disorder, associated neurologic disorders (including cognitive function), hand sensibility, general hand hygiene, ability to voluntarily grasp and release, and the overall severity of the deformity. Zancolli and colleagues recommended various tenotomies and tendon transfers, because they do not believe that wrist arthrodesis is advantageous for such patients [49]. Since that study, however, multiple investigators have recommended complete wrist arthrodesis. Louis and colleagues described a capitate-radius arthrodesis to correct a severely contracted spastic hand [17]. Pomerance and Keenan used wrist arthrodesis as part of a comprehensive single stage corrective procedure that also included superficialis to profundus transfer, wrist flexor tendon release, flexor pollicis longus lengthening, carpal tunnel release, and ulnar motor branch neurectomy or intrinsic release [50]. The surgical indications included failure of conservative management, significant hygiene or nursing care problems, and pain or nerve symptomatology caused by subluxation or compression. The fusion rate was reported to be 87% overall, which is similar to the rates reported for patients with inflammatory, post-traumatic, or degenerative arthritis. Hargreaves and colleagues described a series of 10 patients who had cerebral palsy who underwent 11 complete wrist arthrodeses [51]. A concomitant proximal row carpectomy was performed in eight patients, with soft tissue releases necessary in three patients. Functional improvement was noted in eight wrists, particularly in those patients who had the athetoid pattern. Improvement in hygiene and cosmesis was noted in all of the patients. Alexander and colleagues reported on 18 children who had cerebral palsy who underwent a wrist arthrodesis to correct a severe flexion contracture and ulnar deviation deformity [52]. The mean patient age at the time of surgery was 15.8 years, with an average follow-up of 4.7 years. In 14 of the cases, a proximal row carpectomy also was required. The fusion was stabilized in 16 patients with a one-third tubular or 3.5 DCP plate. The three remaining cases had pin fixation. The mean time to fusion was 3.1 months, and approximately 50% of the patients required subsequent hardware removal for postoperative discomfort. Functional domain outcome studies revealed an average preoperative House score of 1.4 that improved to 3.2 postoperatively. Seventy-two percent of the patients or parents were satisfied with the surgical procedure and they indicated that they would recommend it to others. Significant satisfaction was reported with respect to cosmesis and hygiene.

In general, complete arthrodesis in the pediatric patient can be accomplished successfully with the use of a compression plate regardless of the etiology of the contracture [52–54]. Anderson and Thomas reported on 15 patients who had a flail or partially flail wrist that was fused with an AO-ASIF dynamic compression plate without bone graft [53]. All 15 wrists fused without a major complication at a mean of 11.9 weeks. The investigators reported that stabilization improved the function of the hand and its appearance. Sodl and colleagues reported on the use of a compression plate specifically designed for the pediatric population—the pediatric fusion plate (Synthes USA; Paoli, Pennsylvania) [54]. It is a titanium plate that is 104 mm long with tapering of the plate from 8 mm in width proximally to 6 mm distally. A total of eight screws typically are used. Four 2.7-mm screws are used proximally, and four 2.4-mm screws are inserted distally. The plate is also precontoured in 10° of extension for improved function of the hand.

Patient outcome following wrist arthrodesis

Determination of the functional outcome following a wrist arthrodesis is focused primarily on the amount of pain relief, range of motion of the thumb, fingers, and forearm, ability to perform activities of daily living, ability to return to occupational and avocational activities, and overall patient satisfaction. Early reports relied primarily on the subjective responses of the patient alone and focused on the ability to return to work. Salenius noted that most patients were able to return to heavy manual labor, including automobile and machine fitters [55]. In 1971, Rechnagel reported that 17 of 22 patients who underwent wrist arthrodesis were able to return to work provided that adequate forearm supination and pronation was present [56]. In Hastings and colleagues' series of 89 wrist arthrodeses, 10 patients did not return to work for reasons unrelated to the surgery itself [57]. Of the remaining 79 patients, 51 patients returned to the same preoperative employment activities, 20 patients returned to a less strenuous occupation, and 8 patients were not able to return to work because of reasons related to the wrist.

The ability to return to normal activities of daily living and the same preoperative occupational demands is less clear. Weiss and colleagues reported that patients' subjective assessment of their ability to complete certain tasks indicated that most difficulty was encountered when the wrist was required to be in extreme flexion in a confined space in which the elbow and shoulder could not be used to compensate for the loss of wrist motion [58]. They also stated that activities that required forceful gripping with significant pronation and supination of the forearm were limited also.

Today, more objective measures, including the disabilities of the arm, shoulder, and hand (DASH) and the Buck-Gramcko-Lohman score, are used to determine the success of the procedure. Sauerbier and colleagues used the DASH questionnaire to evaluate those patients who underwent a wrist arthrodesis following Kienbock disease [59]. They reported that 70% of the patients had complete pain relief at rest with 40% pain-free during work conditions. They stated that many patients complained about the reduction in the overall quality of life following the procedure. The successful relief of pain following a wrist arthrodesis seems to be variable according to the literature. O'Bierne and colleagues reported a satisfactory outcome in 81% of their patients following a wrist arthrodesis [60]. In contrast, Sagerman and Palmer noted that all but one of their 17 patients was satisfied with their outcome [61]. Similarly, DeSmet and Truyen reported on 36 patients, 20 of whom had no pain at rest with only 6 patients pain-free during manual activity [62].

A functional assessment of bilateral wrist arthrodeses was performed by Rayan and colleagues, who concluded that most patients maintained a satisfactory functional level postoperatively regarding the activities of daily living, particularly perineal care [63]. They were not able, however, to establish the ideal fusion position for each wrist with respect to optimum function.

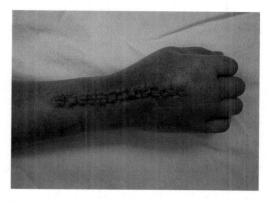

Fig. 5. Postoperative deep wound infection following a wrist arthrodesis in a woman who had a scaphoid nonunion and advanced arthrosis (SNAC wrist).

Complications of complete wrist arthrodesis

Complications following wrist arthrodesis have been described irrespective of the technique used. The complications may be graded as major or minor and include the operative and bone graft donor site. Review of the literature suggests a lower incidence of complications overall with plate fixation [23].

Clendenin and Green reported on a series of 31 patients who underwent wrist arthrodeses using the techniques described by Carroll and Dick, Haddad and Riordan, and Millender and Nalebuff [45]. Major complications were noted in 11 patients, including pseudarthrosis, deep wound infection (Fig. 5), neuroma formation, fracture of a healed fusion, and impingement of the Steinmann pins on the metacarpophalangeal joint. Minor complications occurred in 13 patients, including transient nerve palsy and superficial skin necrosis.

Zachary and Stern reported on 73 wrist arthrodeses in 71 patients using dorsal plate fixation and iliac crest bone graft [64]. Although there was a 100% fusion rate, a total of 82 complications in 50 wrists were encountered. Immediate postoperative wound complications included blistering, significant edema, hematoma formation, and partial dehiscence of the incision. Transient paresthesias in the distribution of the radial, ulnar, and median nerves and postoperative wound infection and significant pain in the region of the DRUJ were also noted. Long-term complications included painful hardware, fracture of the distal radius and third metacarpal, scaphotrapeziotrapezoid (STT) arthritis, metacarpophalangeal joint

stiffness, and long-term neurologic deficit. Approximately 80% of the complications resolved spontaneously or with nonoperative treatment. Surgical treatment was necessary in 19 patients. Resection of the distal ulna was required in three patients and recommended in five others because of symptomatic DRUJ arthritis or ulnar impaction syndrome following the arthrodesis.

Hastings and colleagues reported the results in 89 patients with 90 wrist arthrodeses performed for post-traumatic arthritis [57]. Plate fixation was used in 56 patients (57 wrists) and various other methods were used in the remaining 33 patients (33 wrists). Autogenous iliac crest bone graft was used in all but one of the patients with plate fixation. Nonunion occurred in 2% of the patients with plate fixation and 18% of the patients with an alternative technique. Additional complications occurred in 51% of the patients with plate fixation, compared with 79% of the patients with an alternative technique. Operative treatment was required in 59% of the patients with plate fixation, compared with 21% of the patients with an alternative fixation technique.

Recognized sources of persistent postoperative discomfort and dissatisfaction following an otherwise well performed wrist arthrodesis include DRUJ arthrosis, ulnar impaction syndrome, and carpal tunnel syndrome. These conditions should be assessed carefully preoperatively and addressed at the time of the fusion [23].

Several studies have focused on the specific complications associated with the bone graft donor site [64–66]. Reporting on donor site morbidity following the harvesting of a rib or iliac crest bone graft for maxillofacial reconstruction,

Laurie and colleagues reviewed the results of 104 bone grafts (60 iliac crest and 44 chest) [64]. Rib graft donor site complications included a plural tear, pneumonia, hemothorax, wound dehiscence, chronic pain, and unsightly scarring. Iliac crest donor site complications included prolonged bleeding, hematoma formation, infection, injury to the lateral cutaneous femoral nerve, and prolonged discomfort. In addition, acetabular fracture, unsightly scarring, and an altered gait also were reported. Younger and Chapman reviewed the results in 239 patients with 243 autogenous grafts used for various reconstructive surgical procedures [65]. The overall major complication rate was 8.6%. The specific donor site complications included infection, prolonged wound drainage, hematoma formation, pain lasting longer than 6 months, sensory loss, unsightly scarring, and the need for reoperation. The incidence of minor complications was approximately 21% and included superficial infection, minor wound problems, transient paresthesias, and prolonged donor site discomfort. The morbidity reported with the use of the iliac crest and other alternative donor sites has contributed to the popularity in using cancellous bone graft from the same operative site, specifically the distal radius metaphysis [66].

Summary

Wrist arthrodesis results in a high degree of patient satisfaction and predictable pain relief in most patients. Most patients are able to return to gainful employment, many without impairment. Some patients require restrictions and employment in a less strenuous occupation. Successful fusion rates have been reported in the vast majority of patients overall. Although the functional outcome is acceptable for most patients, some adaptation is necessary, because certain activities such as perineal care and manipulating the hand in tight spaces are difficult. Activities that require forceful gripping with the hand in a fully pronated or supinated position also may be difficult to accomplish. Preoperative counseling of the patient should include a candid discussion of the potential postoperative functional difficulties.

The most common indication for a wrist arthrodesis is advanced symptomatic arthritis secondary to a degenerative, post-traumatic, inflammatory, or postinfectious condition. Wrist arthrodesis also may improve function, hygiene, and cosmesis in the patient who has a contracted or flail wrist associated with cerebral palsy, traumatic brain injury, or brachial plexus injury.

Various techniques have been described for achieving a successful arthrodesis. The type of operative technique used depends on the underlying condition, quality of bone, presence of bilateral disease, condition of the remaining joints of the involved extremity, and surgeon's preference. Intramedullary rod or Steinman pin fixation has been successful in patients who have inflammatory arthritis. Dorsal plate and screw fixation is preferred for patients who have post-traumatic or degenerative arthrosis. Rigid fixation with a dorsal plate is advocated because of the ease of implant application, the high rates of fusion achieved, and the avoidance of prolonged postoperative cast immobilization. Precontoured low profile plates have been developed to position the hand appropriately and to minimize extensor tendon irritation. Controversy still exists as to the ideal position of the hand. Generally the wrist is placed in slight dorsiflexion and ulnar deviation to optimize power grip. In cases of bilateral involvement, the nondominant hand may be placed in 5°–10° of flexion to better assist in such activities as perineal care.

Complications are frequent but can be minimized with attention to detail and good surgical technique. Fortunately most complications are amenable to nonoperative treatment. Major complications include nonunion, deep wound infection, neuroma formation, DRUJ arthritis, ulnocarpal impaction, CTS, and painful retained hardware. Minor complications include hematoma formation, partial wound dehiscence, and transient paresthesias involving the radial, ulnar, or median nerves. Donor site morbidity remains a concern when the iliac crest is used. Complications include hematoma formation, infection, injury to the lateral cutaneous femoral nerve, and prolonged discomfort. Successful outcomes have been reported with the use of local autogenous cancellous bone graft from the distal radius metaphyseal region.

References

[1] Ely LW. A study of joint tuberculosis. Surg Gynecol Obstet 1910;10:561–72.

[2] Ely LW. An operation for tuberculosis of the wrist. JAMA 1920;75(25):1707–9.

[3] Steindler A. Orthopaedic operations on the hand. JAMA 1918;71(10):1288–91.

[4] Stein I. Gill turnabout radial graft for wrist arthrodesis. Surg Gynecol Obstet 1958;106:231–2.

[5] Abbott LC, Saunders JBDM, Bost FC. Arthrodesis of the wrist with the use of grafts of cancellous bone. J Bone Joint Surg 1942;24:883–98.

[6] Colonna PC. A method for fusion of the wrist. South Med J 1944;37:195–9.

[7] Wickstrom JK. Arthrodesis of the wrist. Modification and evaluation of the use of split rib grafts. South Med J 1954;47:968–71.

[8] Evans DL. Wedge arthrodesis of the wrist. J Bone Joint Surg 1955;37:126–34.

[9] Campbell CJ, Keokarn T. Total and subtotal arthrodesis of the wrist. Inlay technique. J Bone Joint Surg 1964;46A:1520–33.

[10] Haddad RJ Jr, Riordan DC. Arthrodesis of the wrist. A surgical technique. J Bone Joint Surg 1967; 49A:950–4.

[11] Clayton ML. Surgical treatment at the wrist in rheumatoid arthritis. A review of thirty-seven patients. J Bone Joint Surg 1965;47A:741–50.

[12] Mannerfelt L, Malmsten M. Arthrodesis of the wrist in rheumatoid arthritis. A technique without external fixation. Scand J Plast Reconstr Surg 1971;5: 124–30.

[13] Larsson SE. Compression arthrodesis of the wrist. A consecutive series of 23 cases. Clin Orthop 1974; 99:146–53.

[14] Bracey DJ, McMurtry RY, Walton D. Arthrodesis in the rheumatoid hand using the AO technique. Orthop Rev 1980;9:65–9.

[15] Wright CS, McMurtry RY. AO arthrodesis in the hand. J Hand Surg [Am] 1983;8:932–5.

[16] Benkeddache Y, Gottesman H, Fourrier P. Multiple stapling for wrist arthrodesis in the nonrheumatoid patient. J Hand Surg [Am] 1984;9:256–60.

[17] Louis DS, Hankin FM, Bowers WH. Capitate-radius arthrodesis: an alternative method of radio-carpal arthrodesis. J Hand Surg [Am] 1984;9: 365–9.

[18] Wood MB. Wrist arthrodesis using dorsal radial bone graft. J Hand Surg [Am] 1987;12:208–12.

[19] Tannenbaum DA, Louis DS. The Stein and Gill technique for wrist arthrodesis. Tech Hand Upper Ext Surg 1999;3(3):181–4.

[20] Voutilainen N, Juutilainen T, Patiala H, et al. Arthrodesis of the wrist with bioabsorbable fixation in patients with rheumatoid arthritis. J Hand Surg [Br] 2002;27:563–7.

[21] Hartigan BJ, Nagle DJ, Foley MJ. Wrist arthrodesis with excision of the proximal carpal bones using the AO/ASIF wrist fusion plate and local bone graft. J Hand Surg [Br] 2001;26(3):247–51.

[22] Meads BM, Scougall PJ, Hargreaves IC. Wrist arthrodesis using a Synthes wrist fusion plate. J Hand Surg [Br] 2003;28(6):571–4.

[23] Jebson PJL, Adams BD. Wrist arthrodesis: review of current techniques. J Am Acad Orthop Surg 2001; 9(1):53–60.

[24] Szabo RM, Thorson EP, Raskind JR. Allograft replacement with distal radioulnar joint fusion and ulnar osteotomy for treatment of giant cell tumors of the distal radius. J Hand Surg 1990;15A:929–33.

[25] Brumfield RH, Champoux JA. A biomechanical study of normal functional wrist motion. Clin Orthop 1984;187:23–5.

[26] Rayan GM, Brentlinger A, Purnell D, et al. Functional assessment of bilateral wrist arthrodeses. J Hand Surg [Am] 1987;12:1020–4.

[27] Clayton ML, Ferlic DC. Arthrodesis of the arthritic wrist. Clin Orthop 1984;187:89–93.

[28] Ilian DI, Rettig ME. Rheumatoid arthritis of the wrist. Bull Hosp Joint Dis 2003;61(3–4):179–85.

[29] Taleisnik J. Rheumatoid arthritis of the wrist. Hand Clin 1989;5(2):257–78.

[30] Dupont M, Vainio K. Arthrodesis of the wrist in rheumatoid arthritis. A study of 140 cases. Ann Chir Gynaecol Fenn 1968;57(4):513–9.

[31] Carroll RE, Dick HM. Arthrodesis of the wrist for rheumatoid arthritis. J Bone Joint Surg 1971;53A: 1365–9.

[32] Shapiro JS. The wrist in rheumatoid arthritis. Hand Clin 1996;12(3):477–98.

[33] Lorei MP, Figgie MP, Ranawat CS, et al. Failed total wrist arthroplasty. Analysis of failures and results of operative management. Clin Orthop Rel Res 1997;34(2):84–93.

[34] Beer TA, Turner RH. Wrist arthrodesis for failed implant arthroplasty. J Hand Surg 1997;22(4): 685–93.

[35] Millender LH, Nalebuff EA. Arthrodesis of the rheumatoid wrist. An evaluation of sixty patients and a description of a different surgical technique. J Bone Joint Surg 1973;55(5):1026–34.

[36] Mikkelsen OA. Arthrodesis of the wrist joint in rheumatoid arthritis. Hand 1980;12(2):149–53.

[37] Papaioannou T, Dickson RA. Arthrodesis of the wrist in rheumatoid disease. Hand 1982;14(1): 12–6.

[38] Mohty A, Hassan D, Shapiro S, Green DL. An alternative technique for revision arthrodesis of the rheumatoid wrist: a case report. J Hand Surg 2001;26(1): 105–8.

[39] Masada K, Yasuda M, Takeuchi E, et al. Technique of intra-medullary fixation for arthrodesis of the wrist in rheumatoid arthritis. Scand J Plast Reconstr Surg 2003;37(3):155–8.

[40] Straub LR, Ranawat CS. The wrist in rheumatoid arthritis. Surgical treatment and results. J Bone Joint Surg 1969;51(1):1–20.

[41] Weiss APC. Osteoarthritis of the wrist. Instr Course Lect 2004;53:31–40.

[42] Adams BD. Surgical management of the arthritic wrist. Inst Course Lect 2004;53:41–5.

[43] Divelbiss BJ, Baratz ME. The role of arthroplasty and arthrodesis following trauma to the upper extremity. Hand Clin 1999;15(2):335–45.

[44] Freeland AE, Sud V, Jemison DM. Early wrist arthrodesis for irreparable intra-articular distal radial fractures. J Hand Surg 2000;5(2):113–8.

[45] Clendenin MB, Green DP. Arthrodesis of the wrist—complications and their management. J Hand Surg 1981;6(3):253–7.

[46] Corfield L, Hampton R, McCullough CJ. Wrist arthrodesis following ulnar bar excision in fibrodysplasia ossificans progressiva. J Hand Surg [Br] 2000; 25(2):223–4.

[47] Epstein S. Arthrodesis for flail wrist. Am J Surg 1930;8(3):622.

[48] Nissen KI. Symposium on cerebral palsy (orthopaedic section). J R Soc Med 1951;44:87–90.

[49] Zancolli EA, Goldner LJ, Swanson AB. Surgery of the spastic hand in cerebral palsy: report of committee on spastic evaluation. J Hand Surg 1983;8(5): 766–72.

[50] Pomerance JF, Keenan MAE. Correction of severe spastic flexion contractures in the non-functional hand. J Hand Surg 1996;21(5):828–33.

[51] Hargreaves DG, Warwick DJ, Tomkin MA. Changes in hand function following wrist arthrodesis in cerebral palsy. J Hand Surg [Br] 2000;25(2):193–4.

[52] Alexander RD, Davids JR, Crower-Peace LC, et al. Wrist arthrodesis in children with cerebral palsy. J Ped Orthop 2000;20(4):490–5.

[53] Anderson GA, Thomas BP. Arthrodesis of flail or partially flail wrists using a dynamic compression plate without bone grafting. J Bone Joint Surg [Br] 2000;82(4):566–70.

[54] Sodl JF, Kozin SH, Kaufmann RA. Development and use of a wrist fusion plate for children and adolescents. J Ped Ortho 2002;22(2):146–9.

[55] Salenius P. Arthrodesis of the carpal joint. Acta Orthop Scand 1966;37(3):288–96.

[56] Rechnagel K. Arthrodesis of the wrist joint. A follow-up of sixty cases. Scand J Plast Reconstr Surg 1971;5(2):120–3.

[57] Hastings H II, Weiss APC, Quenzer D, et al. Arthrodesis of the wrist for post-traumatic disorders. J Bone Joint Surg 1996;78(6):897–902.

[58] Weiss APC, Hastings H. Wrist arthrodesis for traumatic conditions: a study of plate and local bone graft application. J Hand Surg 1995;20(1):50–6.

[59] Sauerbier M, Kluge S, Bickert B, et al. Subjective and objective outcomes after total wrist arthrodesis in patients with radiocarpal arthrosis or Kienböck's disease. Chir Main 2000;19(4):223–31.

[60] O'Bierne J, Boyer MI, Axelrod TS. Wrist arthrodesis using a dynamic compression plate. J Bone Joint Surg Br 1995;77(5):700–4.

[61] Sagerman SD, Palmer AK. Wrist arthrodesis using a dynamic compression plate. J Hand Surg [Br] 1996;21(4):437–41.

[62] De Smet L, Truyen J. Arthrodesis of the wrist for osteoarthritis: outcome with a minimum follow-up of 4 years. J Hand Surg [Br] 2003;28(6):575–7.

[63] Zachary SV, Stern PJ. Complications following AO/ASIF wrist arthrodesis. J Hand Surg [Am] 1995; 20(2):339–44.

[64] Laurie SW, Kaban LB, Mulliken JB, et al. Donor-site morbidity after harvesting rib and iliac bone. Plast Reconstr Surg 1984;73(6):933–8.

[65] Younger EM, Chapman MW. Morbidity at bone graft donor sites. J Orthop Trauma 1989;3(3):192–5.

[66] Weiss APC, Wiedeman G, Quenzer D, et al. Upper extremity function after wrist arthrodesis. J Hand Surg [Am] 1995;20A:813–7.

ELSEVIER
SAUNDERS

Hand Clin 21 (2005) 641–654

HAND
CLINICS

Cumulative Index 2005

Note: Page numbers of article titles are in **boldface** type.

0749-0712/05/$ - see front matter © 2005 Elsevier Inc. All rights reserved.
doi:10.1016/S0749-0712(05)00106-X

hand.theclinics.com